BEECHCROFT LLC
SLEEP AND
DREAM RESEARCH

Research and Education Association
505 Eighth Avenue
New York, N. Y. 10018

SLEEP AND DREAM RESEARCH

Printed in the United States of America

Library of Congress Catalog Card Number 82-62130

International Standard Book Number 0-87891-545-1

Preface

This book reports on the studies of sleep which have provided unforeseen insights into human behavior. The convergence of efforts by many researchers has resulted in the rapid development of new techniques and practical knowledge — especially with regard to the brain's activity.

The exploration of sleep is relatively new, but it has already contributed towards (1) understanding infant development, (2) an understanding of the effects of drugs and the development of more sensitive drug therapy, and (3) the clinical diagnosis and treatment of a variety of mental disorders — sleep disorders are characteristic of many mental illnesses.

The information in this book was originated and sponsored by the National Institute of Mental Health.

Table of Contents

Chapter I.
Clocks Within the Body

Before electricity, light was precious, difficult to produce and expensive to buy, and most of the human world retired when darkness fell. The custom of sleeping through the night probably stems from the long history of necessity. Perhaps nightly sleep, or at least the general habit of mankind of sleeping many hours at one stretch, is the stamp of this history upon the organization of our bodies.

Insofar as we know, people the world over sleep between 5 and 8 hours at a stretch, usually at night. If this were sheer custom one might expect to hear about cultures with other habits, perhaps places where naps constituted the entire sleep of people, places where sleep was equally apportioned as are our three meals a day. Such cultures may somewhere exist, but they have not been reported.

In Spain and many Latin countries, of course, there is the custom of the afternoon siesta, a long nap. Nevertheless, people in these countries sleep some 5–7 hours again at night. A visitor to Bali has claimed that the Balinese do not sleep all night, for they sing when they are awake and there is no time of day or night when singing cannot be heard in the villages. Unfortunately, such anecdotal reporting inspires faulty conclusions. Casual reports from tourists once suggested that the northern Norwegians slept remarkably little during the summer. Travelers had made this inference after cruises along the coast, for in this season of the midnight sun there were always townspeople along the docks, whatever the time of day or night. However, the conclusion was negated by Dr. Nathaniel Kleitman, a physiologist whose systematic studies of sleep have provided inspiration for much of the current work. Kleitman and his daughter interviewed the townspeople of Tromso, in that northern coastal region, and found that they slept about 7 hours a day in the summer and only an hour longer in the winter. Other Arctic studies offer about the same figures, emphasizing that man's sleep is not solely determined by light and dark (Kleitman and Kleitman, 1953; Semagin, 1961).

Social customs and the organization of work and rest are oriented around light and dark throughout the world, and nightly sleep is the predominant pattern. This appears to be changing somewhat in urban societies, where some industries and professions demand night work, portending a 24-hour operation. The data processing center in Rockefeller Plaza, for instance, is in constant operation as are newspapers, radio, TV, creating professions to which many night people, so called, are attracted. Many people in urban centers appear to prefer night activity and

2

day-long sleep. Ferenc Molnar, the playwright, was so extreme in this respect he is said to have seen daylight only on a rare occasion. There is a story that he had to appear in court as a witness one morning, and as friends taxied him into town about an hour after his normal retiring time, Molnar blearily looked out at the springtime streets of Budapest and could not believe that so many people would be up and about. "Are they all witnesses?" he wanted to know.

Although not every one does his sleeping at night, everyone, it appears, sleeps for a long interval once in every 24 hours. We do not know whether there is any intrinsic need to sleep many hours at a stretch, or whether we require some absolute amount of sleep that might be differently apportioned. Until other practices are found among human cultures or demonstrated in the laboratory, we have reason to assume that our sleep schedule is interknit with a system of physiological periods that revolve, like the earth, around an axis of 24 hours. The survival of a species is served by rhythms, biological clocks that are adapted to nature's periodicities. Such rhythms are found in all forms of life and seem to be among their most basic characteristics (Kleitman, 1963; Murray, in press; Richter, 1965). Although they are usually related to cycles in the environment, such as light and dark, they will persist for long periods even in the absence of such environmental change. The morning-glory is known to every child for blooming by day and closing at night. Similarly, algae, insects, and vertebrate creatures have inbuilt cycles. The owl and the bat are nocturnal, but most higher mammals are diurnal, sleeping in darkness and waking in light (Berlucchi and Strata, 1962). Man is no exception to this internal patterning.

There may be a relatively simple explanation for the nocturnal activity of some animal species. The cat is such an animal, and something is known about the mechanism in the cat. His nervous system appears to be directly responsive to darkness. A sensory apparatus within the eye dispatches neural impulses when light stimulation stops (Arduini and Pinneo, 1962, 1963). This is known as the dark discharge of the retina. Dr. A. Arduini and his coworkers at the University of Pisa have shown that this dark discharge has an arousing effect upon the cat. If other conditions remain constant the cat is more likely to be awake and alert during darkness, and this phenomenon has been shown to be due to dark discharge from the retina. By eliminating the dark discharge from the retina in laboratory studies, the experimental cats were prevented from showing their natural tendency to come alert during darkness.

This connection, which has been established experimentally between the dak-sensitive retina of the cat's eye and the creature's arousal system in the base of its brain, helps to explain a cat's preference for night prowling. There is now a growing literature on such cyclical mechanisms as oxygen metabolism in simple organisms, and biological clocks within many forms of life, but in the higher organisms there are many internal rhythms. Within the human body it is safe to assume that there is a constant interplay of different cycles, whose time periods and effects upon our lives fall beyond the scope of present knowledge.

Cycles and Illness

Man's days, his nights, his diseases, his times of trouble, periods of confusion, moments of clarity, may well be determined and balanced by a delicate and vastly complex intermeshing of biological time cycles. We are accustomed to recognizing the most obvious and predictable periods—infancy, childhood, maturation, and old age—although we know little about the mechanisms that make this schedule of life so predictable. Some internal cycles, like the 28-day menstrual cycle are well known; however, the individual pays little attention to most of his physiological cycles, indeed remains unaware that his fluctuations are periodic. Dr. Curt Richter of Johns Hopkins observed that many uncommon physical disorders follow odd periodicities ranging from 48 hours to 17 months. There are other illnesses whose symptoms rise and fall in cycles of 7 days or 52 days. Such ailments as swelling of the knee, certain lymph disorders and psychoses appear to grow acute in a periodic fashion (Richter, 1965). Richter has speculated—an hypothesis we are not now capable of confirming—that the body's many metabolisms have particular cycles of activity, and that these are generally out of phase so that the system as a whole is rather constant. But shock, emotional trauma, or allergic shock might so jar the system that some of these components become synchronized, causing the whole system to wax and wane in phase with them—with amplified effects known as illness. Although this is a very empyrean speculation at the

5

moment, it may prove pertinent when we are able to tamper seriously with man's sleep cycles, and it may suggest some long-term links in the etiology of sleep disorder and mental disease, for the two are commonly associated.

The Circadian Rhythm

Although biological periodicities may play a very large role in our lives, we are influenced by them unaware, and have done little to utilize any but the most gross periods for our benefit. Most people do not realize that their body temperature varies rhythmically about a degree or two every day. This circadian temperature rhythm (from the Latin "circa dies," meaning about a day) exists after about the third month of life, perhaps inherited from the mother's cycle. With almost clocklike regularity the body temperature rises and falls each 24 hours. The highest temperature is likely to coincide with a person's "best hours" of wakefulness, his favorite time of day, the time when he feels most alive and alert. The nadir generally occurs in the late hours of sleep. If a person happens to be awake during this low-temperature period he may sense a slump in his vitality and may feel chilled. The high temperature period is associated with the muscular tension we exhibit when awake and the low temperature is associated with the relaxation of our muscles during sleep, but the cause of the temperature cycle is unknown. It may result from an intermeshing of many metabolic periodicities. Whatever its origins, the circadian temperature cycle appears to be quite hard to alter in the normal adult.

One of the most famous attempts to shift from

a 24-hour cycle to another schedule took place in Mammoth Cave, Ky., in June 1938. Nathaniel Kleitman and a student descended into a chamber of cool and unchanging temperature, where silence was unbroken, darkness absolute but for electric light. There, in a cave usually traversed by tourists, they set up living quarters and tried to shuck the 24-hour day. They were not shooting for extreme changes—just a 21-hour day and a 28-hour day. It seemed easier to compress the cycle than to stretch it. Kleitman, then in his early forties, found that he adapted less easily than the younger man. When he tried to follow the sleep schedule of a 6-day week (a 28-hour day) his body stubbornly showed the temperature cycle of a 7-day week. Although a group of explorers reported following a 21- and 27-hour day in the arctic summer, nobody has ever managed a 30- or 48-hour day. The 24-hour temperature cycle tends to resist radical modification insofar as we know (Kleitman, 1963).

We know very little about the fluctuations in body chemistry that accompany this regular rise and fall of temperature. The adrenal glands produce hormones whose concentration in the urine follows the same rise and fall as body temperature. Similarly, the concentration of eosinophils in the blood mirror the 24-hour cycle: these are a special type of white blood cell produced in bone marrow. Presumably an interlocking of many metabolic elements is involved. New information on the circadian temperature rhythm, diurnal sleep cycle, and body chemistry may come from attempts to develop a drug that lowers man's body temperature

7

and oxygen consumption, putting him into a state comparable to sleep. A drug induced hibernation, so to speak, might entail a drastic alteration in the circadian rhythm and has many possible applications if the trick can be performed without injury.

At present, however, we have had notably little success in expanding or contracting the cycle in adult animals. Using environmental change it has been possible to modify cycles in termites, crustaceans, and invertebrates, hardly tantamount to altering the circadian rhythm in higher mammals, but we are meanwhile learning a good deal about rhythms by shifting the phase of the daily cycle—so that the peak and nadir temperatures, while in the same relation to each other, occur at a different time than normally.

Man and his cousin primates are the only animals with very pronounced diurnal cycles, waking by day, sleeping through the night. Macaque and rhesus monkeys are typically active for 12–16 hours, and then lapse into a long period of inactivity (Rhodes, 1964; Weitzman et al., 1964). In one effort to discover the controlling factors in this cycle three infant monkeys were raised in a constant environment, always dark excepting for 1 hour of diffuse light each day. The monkeys were put on different feeding and light schedules for periods of 3–5 weeks. Changes in feeding time did not affect the monkeys, but when the daily hour of light was shifted, the animals would slowly show an activity cycle that stabilized around the time of the light. Light seemed to have a greater impact on their daily fluctuations than did food (Lindsley et al., 1962).

8

Light evidently affects the nervous system and physiological function in profound ways that we are just beginning to uncover (Lisk et al., 1965). In many mammals, for instance, light enhances pituitary-gonadal functioning. Direct light to hypothalamus, shone through implanted tubes, has produced in rats a continuous estrouslike cycle, with a rise in ovarian weight and pituitary weight. In ducks, other studies have shown that direct light to certain brain regions stimulated the gonads. Thus, light itself affects the central nervous system so as to influence steroid production, thereby influencing reproduction. Not all of the physiologically influential light need be coming through the eyes. Sunlight, it has been shown, can penetrate the hypothalamus of sheep, dog, rabbit, and rat, perhaps in this way affecting the periods known as breeding seasons.

Cycles and Medicine

Despite the existence of night people and the fact that we have no clear understanding of the role of light in our diurnal rhythm, it is possible that light affects our nervous systems in such a way as to orient our circadian rhythm—acting as an entraining agent. Because it has this effect upon lower animals, experimentalists have used illumination schedules to stabilize the circadian rhythm in studies that may have vast implications for human welfare. Our temperature cycles and subcycles may exert a powerful influence on our behavior, attention shifts, ability to work, response to illness, even our capacity to survive. Hospital personnel, for instance, make the casual observation that the predawn hours are often the fatal ones for critically ill people. They are a time of many coronaries. Is there a correlation between events in the temperature cycle of patients and their time of death (Snyder et al., 1964)? If the low temperature period coincides with the time of symptom intensity and crisis, one might expect the people who work all night to show a crisis tendency that falls at quite different hours than people who work by day. Animal experiments suggest that there are regular low activity periods and these may indeed be intervals of physiological vulnerability.

Experiments on rats have indicated that the animals are particularly vulnerable to the botulinus bacillus during their inactive periods, so differentially sensitive that the time of injection may determine whether there is acute illness, like that of food poisoning, or death. The daily rhythmicity appears to pervade the metabolic system, and animal studies have shown up differential responsivity to temperature, ultraviolet light, and drugs. Within the laboratory an artificial lighting regimen can help to stabilize the phase orientation of the animals' temperature cycles. When maintained on light for the 12 hour period between 7 a.m. and 7 p.m., and dark the remaining hours, two strains of mice showed particular vulnerability to X-radiation when the dosage was administered at midnight, 19 hours after the beginning of the light cycle. The survival of mice after high-intensity irradiation was, in a series of studies, demonstrably responsive to the different phase points on the daily temperature cycle. The effect of X-radiation during the animal's subjective night was far worse than during subjective day. After radiation all the mice became very sick, but those irradiated at 9 a.m. eventually recovered, whereas those irradiated at 9 p.m. did not recover. Those irradiated between midnight and 4 a.m. were maximally vulnerable. At high, almost lethal dosages, the animals had some chance of surviving X-radiation if it occurred during certain phases of their circadian cycle, but their chances diminished at other points on the cycle, and they were doomed if it occurred at their interval of greatest sensitivity (Pizzarello et al., 1964).

Judging from animal studies, and from the very fabric of the language in which man describes subjective waxing and waning of strength, it would seem that the circadian temperature cycle holds many implications for understanding behavior and illness, and for the timing of treatments. If, indeed, most patients are highly vulnerable during the dawn and early morning hours, some changes in hospital schedules might be warranted. During the past year a reported discussion among medical doctors suggested that surgery should not be scheduled too early in the morning if possible and that the traditional hospital regimen may disturb patients too early. At this point there are no organized data on the relative merits of timing hospital procedures or clinic treatments differently, and until recently there has been no reasonable way of obtaining continuous body-temperature readings from acutely ill patients without disturbing them. Procedures for using very small thermistors are being developed in several places, among them the Downstate Medical Center in

New York. Statistical information about the influence of man's temperature cycle may generate means of gauging an individual's inner timing, periods of strength and weakness, and may also help us to understand the effect of this daily cycle upon the performance of people at work, upon emotional fluctuations, and the ability to withstand stress. The temperature cycle may also hold useful clues to the timing of symptoms in disease and mental disorder.

Cycles and Work Schedules

At present, the working world abides by a clock into which individuals must fit as best they can. Although it may be of considerable practical consequence to us we know very little about the interaction of the circadian temperature rhythm with the external schedule. Researches inspired by different aims suggest that temperature cycles may offer valuable guidelines by which people could perform at their best and avoid performing at their worst if they scheduled their most demanding work for periods of higher temperature and avoided commitments during the interval of their nadir (Loveland and Williams; Williams, Lubin, and Goodnow; Wilkinson, in press; Alluisi, et al.; Murray, et al., 1958). In the course of a somewhat repetitive daily schedule, people do undoubtedly orient themselves more-or-less according to their cycle. However, rapid communications, jet travel, and requirements for round-the-clock productivity are becoming more common, are disrupting the regularity of the work schedule, and demanding greater flexibility of many people. Surely, space travel will impose round-the-clock demands upon the first venturers, and in looking forward to these a number of studies have been made on men who performed various kinds of tasks in enclosed chambers. Dr. E. A. Alluisi and his associates have shown that a man's efficiency can be diminished during a decline of temperature if the situation forces him to handle an appreciable increment in information.

In a series of studies sponsored by the Air Force, different work-rest schedules have been tried out on selected volunteers for periods of 10 days to a month (Ray, et al., 1961). What are the merits of working for 4 hours and then resting for 2 hours? What ratio of work and rest permits a man to be most productive over a period of time? Such questions are difficult to answer and may depend in part upon the nature of the job. In one study a group of highly motivated cadets was cooped up in a small crew compartment for 15 days, with taxing jobs to do, such as picking out radar "target" signals from a noisy screen. The special attribute of these tasks was that they were entirely dependent upon the individual whereas other similar confinement studies placed emphasis upon group cooperation (Passey, et al., 1964). As the experimenters varied the task requirements and schedules of work and sleep, they observed that a highly motivated young cadet could work a 16-hour day (on duty for 4 hours and off duty for 2 hours) more easily than a lighter day (of 4 hours duty and 4 hours rest), but only under some conditions. Surely, for the purposes of a sensitive and costly mission like a space flight, the best schedule ought to enable a man to remain very steady in his performance and not render him unduly vulnerable to stresses such as sleep loss. Alluisi and his coworkers have found that a short period of sleep loss seems to reveal the practicality or performance endurance of work-rest schedules. By using a 48-hour period of sleep deprivation, they have found that performance is far more uneven on a 4–2 schedule than on a schedule of 4-hour duty and 4-hour rest. The stress of sleep loss has been used as a means of distinguishing between schedules.

Some scientific questions raised by the prospect of space flight should lead to research which, in turn, should reveal more information about the nature of our circadian cycle and its influence in our lives, information that would be of immense practical value. We do not now know what would happen to an individual if he were placed in a timeless, unchanging environment, a place of no clocks, no mealtimes, no schedule, and no change in light. Would his diurnal cycle begin to fragment? Would he sleep in short intervals like a young baby? How would his health and work capacity be affected? We do not know how much the biological clocks inside are meshed with an external environment. These questions are intimately linked with man's patterns of sleep and with the possible means and consequences of changing sleep patterns (McKenzie, et al., 1960).

A number of scientists have speculated that sleep—as we indulge in it—may be a habit and that the circadian temperature rhythm, with the many metabolic systems implied, could be altered by training in infancy. A lifelong habit, like sleeping 8 hours each night, has a profound physical meaning, for it becomes imbedded in the organization of the central nervous system, in the biochemical timing of the body, and the word "habit" should not imply that this is a pattern that can be changed easily, if at all. However profound its effects, there is still evidence that training plays a greater role in human behavior than it does in lower animals. There are now studies underway, of humans and of animals, that may elucidate the role of habit in our sleep patterns and circadian rhythm.

An initial survey of some 600 people was undertaken by the Gainesville, Fla., laboratory directed by Dr. Wilse B. Webb. Intensive questionnaires were issued to men, women, and children of different ages in the hope of amassing some gross statistics about the role of training, such as the possibility that family sleep patterns are consistent among family members. Do early-rising parents train their children to be early risers throughout life? Another approach being considered in several laboratories is that of forcing unusual sleep and waking schedules upon infant animals. If early training were a large factor, it might be possible to alter the circadian rhythm in animals and, perhaps, man. This might be convenient for man in the coming decades as artificial light, rapid travel, and unusual tasks alter the routine that was once bounded by natural day and night.

Light and darkness, distance and time have converged for modern man, and especially today individuals could benefit from a greater sensitivity to their own daily rhythms and an understanding of their relation to performance. Nobody doubts that there is really a difference between the early riser, the so-called lark, and the night owl stereotype. Yet, recognizing the great range in sleep-waking preferences, we still fail to concede that they are of much importance. The rigidity or flexibility of a person's sleep habits may be a result of early training, for instance, and information on this point alone could be valuable in rearing future generations. However, unless a person is stricken with an illness like encephalitis, his circadian rhythm remains, and his body temperature will rise and fall on a 24-hour schedule. It is not even easy to shift the phase of this cycle very rapidly, a basis for the complaints of some travelers. These days it is not uncommon for a business executive to leave his office shortly before noon, for instance, and fly as far from New York to Honolulu to direct an after-dinner meeting. As he speaks at what is 8 p.m. for the Hawaiians, it is 1 a.m. New York time, and by the time the question period is over his weary body decrees that it is 3 a.m., however early the clocks read in Honolulu. Individuals react very differently to a life in which such time-shifts are frequent, and there is no saying what impact such a schedule may have upon their health and performance.

For many practical purposes—medicine, industry, and perhaps particularly preventive medicine—a further investigation of the circadian rhythm and its relationship with the environment will be extremely useful. Further explorations should reveal something about the nature of the subcycles that are reflected in small fluctuations in body temperature, and perhaps determine the fluctuations that people report in their abilities to concentrate, the waxing and waning of attention, fluctuations of about 90–120 minutes that appear to take place throughout the day and night.

One cannot say that the circadian rhythm is the reason that man sleeps for long periods, usually at night, or that it is totally inelastic, but there is strong evidence that it is related to our patterns of sleep and that it is composed of subcycles. The study of biological rhythms in man promises to yield information of practical and medical value, perhaps enabling clinicians to utilize optimum timing as part of treatment. If subcycles of the daily rhythm influence our waxing and waning of waking attention and mood, we may learn how they bear on waking activity through the study of sleep—for a night of sleep itself consists of recurrent cycles of brain activity and physiological change.

Chapter II.
A Night of Sleep

Each night at an accustomed time people begin to set the stage for sleep with small rituals that lead to bed and darkness. A dusk of consciousness will fall like a curtain on the day and soon, from outside, the body will seem still but for a shallow and even breathing. A twisting, a groan, fluttering of eyelids and perhaps muffled sounds may occasionally break the stillness, but for 7 or 8 hours the person seems to have departed, gone from the world into a silent internal communion from which he will rise like an amnesic. The forgetting, the sense of oblivion is so nearly complete that it is surprising how easily people accept this suspension from life, relinquishing themselves each night with little anxiety. Primitive people, understandably enough, often looked upon sleep as a temporary death, and remnants of their uncertainty and fear can be found in religious liturgies; one example is an Orthodox Jewish morning prayer, thanking the Lord for the return of the soul and therefore life. Although the sleeper is clearly animate, his prolonged stillness scarcely conveys to an observer any sense of the tides within.

Sleep, as we now know it, is not a state of unconsciousness, an oblivion punctuated by occasional dreams. It is not, indeed, a unitary state of being, but a progression of rhythmic cycles representing different phases of neural function. By watching a person sleep, the observer cannot see that the sleeper is rising and falling on the waves of a recurrent tide. Nor can he observe that the sleeper regularly enters long intervals so different from the rest of sleep that some scientists have called it another state—a state of frenzied internal activity, resembling in many ways alert wakefulness. The bedside observer cannot easily detect the signs of shifts within, for the place to watch a night of sleep is not in the bedroom—but in the recordings of laboratory polygraphs, the electroencephalograph, the cardiogram, myograph, and thermometer.

The Electroencephalograph

The progression of cycles that make up a night's sleep have been pieced together by numerous observers through nightlong vigils in sleep laboratories. There are perhaps 2 dozen sleep laboratories in the United States, in university buildings and hospitals. They vary somewhat in size and newness, and complexity of equipment, but laboratories designed for the study of human sleep basically resemble each other. In the control room the visitor will notice the fundamental polygraph instruments, consolidated in the big amplifier system, the electroencephalograph machine, a device through which researchers can watch brain activity. Small conductive electrodes, bits of metal pasted onto the scalp, or in some cases, needles implanted in the brain, transmit the natural beat of a brain region through changes of electric potential. The electroencephalograph (EEG) amplifies these shifts in potential, transmitting them to magnetic tape, or driving a row of ink pens on the desklike panel of the machine. Each pen, driven by a signal from a part of the brain, moves up when the electric charge is negative and down when the charge becomes positive. As a continuous sheet of graph paper moves forward on a roller, at a constant speed, under the oscillating pens, the up-and-down pen movements are traced out as waves—brain waves. Their amplitude indicates the ever shifting amount of voltage generated in a brain region, and their shape can indicate the speed of the electrical changes within. Thus, a glance at the inked record will tell whether the potentials in the brain are shifting in a regular, synchronous fashion, with slow, large voltage changes, or whether the changes are fast and irregular, desynchronized.

Although some body functions can be detected by simply looking at a person, precise and reliable measures of blood pressure, pulse, respiration, muscle tone, temperature require sensing devices that can produce signals to be amplified and recorded in the manner of brain waves. In order to minimize interference with sleep, researchers now use some of the miniature instruments developed for space exploration. For example, a thermistor no bigger than a pin can be used to detect body temperature continuously. This kind of equipment enables simultaneous recordings of heart rate and temperature fluctuations on the same record as the EEG, showing how changes in brain wave patterns are related to changing body functions.

The Sleep Laboratory

On any evening, when most people have settled down to an after-dinner entertainment or are preparing for bed, the sleep scientist has begun to check out his equipment. Inkwells are filled, pens cleaned, wire leads tested for insulation and possible breaks, and a thousand-foot sheet of folded EEG paper inserted between the rollers, reels of magnetic tape set in place. Continual adjustments, requiring some manual and electronic dexterity, are essential to reliable data collection, and before the arrival of a sleep subject, the control room resembles the cockpit of a plane during the instrument check for takeoff.

The aura of the sleep laboratory is similar, whether it is 10-below-zero on the snowbound University of Chicago campus where a solitary row of lights mark the brownstone containing the laboratory, or a balmy California night outside the vast and silent new hospital at UCLA. The sleep researcher collects his data largely during these lonely hours, a strenuous pursuit, sometimes requiring vigils for many consecutive nights, weeks, or even months. It is an endeavor requiring physical and mental endurance, one that places a strain on all personal or social activity, for it may be necessary to monitor the sleep of others on many consecutive nights while fulfilling administrative and academic duties and analyzing the data by day.

Our current picture of a night's sleep is a composite of thousands of nights and thousands of volunteers, most of them young men in their twenties, generally students or professionals. Very often they are paid a small sum to sleep in the laboratory and abide by the rules of the study—which may prohibit napping, drinking coffee or alcohol, and taking drugs. Typically, the young volunteer will arrive before 10 p.m., change into pajamas, and seat himself in some corner of the laboratory to be decorated for the night.

Often, in the strong odor of acetone and collodion, used to fasten electrodes to the skin, the experimenter will conduct a quiet and soothing conversation as he carefully affixes the electrodes to the top of the head, at the temples, near the eyes. Each electrode disc has a brightly colored lead, following a color code, and the many-colored wires are often drawn through a ring at the top of the head like a pigtail. When the preparation is securely finished, the volunteer will go to bed in one of the quiet bedrooms adjacent to the control room. The room is ordinary enough, except for a jackboard at the head of the bed, and an intercom system. The wires from the volunteer's head are plugged into the jack-board, and he settles down. The lights go out. The bed is comfortable, and the volunteer can move freely, although he cannot get up and walk around ordinarily without being unplugged. If he wants anything, however, he can tell the experimenter through the intercom system.

The room is private, the volunteer is comfortable, the technical details of the study well in hand,

and one might expect that data collection would be quite routine. In all human studies, however, there is an emotional component, and the somewhat predictable, somewhat elusive interplay of feelings adds a heavy burden to the sleep study. Even a well-balanced medical student may have a hard time falling asleep in his private bedroom although accustomed to being in laboratories; the gentlemen beyond the door are monitoring his brain waves, and although he knows that EEG patterns do not invade mental privacy in the sense that they cannot reveal thought or dream content, the laboratory situation is strange.

"The Laboratory Effect"

On their first night subjects often do not exhibit the sleep patterns that seem characteristic of them on later nights. A night or two of adjustment may be necessary, in full headdress. Sometimes as many as five or more consecutive nights will be necessary to obtain the baseline—the usual pattern of the individual's sleep—before the experimenter collects a sole night of data (Dement, Greenberg, and Klein, 1965). However trivial the bias may be in a particular study, and no matter what precautions have been taken, the so-called "laboratory effect" resides within all the generalizations being drawn from human studies—as illustrated by the fact that among hundreds of young men in the laboratories, nightmares and wet dreams have been extremely rare. Thus, in speaking of the typical night of sleep as we now see it, we must bear in mind some modifications for it is a composite of nights spent in a laboratory.

Drowsiness

Usually, about 11 p.m., the acclimated volunteer will be relaxed. His body temperature is declining. His eyes are closed, and he is no longer moving. On the graph paper in the control room the jumble of rapid, irregular brain waves is beginning to form a new pattern, a regular rhythm known as the alpha rhythm. This pattern of 9–12 cycles a second indicates relaxed wakefulness. Subjectively, it is a serene and pleasant state, devoid of deliberate thought, into which images may float. A moment of tension or attempt to solve a mental proble will disrupt it (Kamiya, 1962).

With further relaxation the alpha waves grow smaller, decreasing in amplitude. As alpha rhythm diminishes, a person's time perception seems to deteriorate, and two rapid flashes of light may seem to blend into one (Anliker, 1963). As his alpha rhythm diminishes, the young volunteer hovers on the borders of drowsiness and sleep, perhaps seeing images, experiencing d r e a m l i k e thoughts or fragments (Foulkes and Vogel).

Stage 1

Another pattern begins to emerge on the EEG paper. This new script is smaller, indicating lower voltages. It is uneven, desynchronized, and it changes swiftly. At this point one may experience a floating sensation, drifting with idle images as the alpha rhythm gives way to the low voltage, fast irregular rhythm of the first stage of sleep. (Kamiya, 1961; Foulkes and Vogel). The volunteer, in this phase, can be easily awakened by a noise or spoken word. His body muscles are relaxing. Respiration is growing more even and heart rate is becoming slower (Snyder, 1960). If awakened at this point a person may assert that he was not really asleep. This phase of consciousness is like a port of entry, a borderland, and lasts only a few minutes. Soon the background rhythm of the EEG grows slower.

Stage 2

The script grows larger and the pens trace out quick bursts known as spindles, rapid crescendos and decrescendos of waves. The eyes of the young volunteer may appear to be slowly rolling. He is quite soundly asleep, yet it is not hard to awaken him. By now there has been a fundamental change in his brain function. One aspect of this change is suggested by a study in which volunteers slept with their eyes half open; illuminated objects were suspended before their eyes. On the whole they were not awakened by the light, nor did they remember seeing anything, but when awakened by a voice a few seconds later they often insisted they had been wide awake and thinking thoughts that, as narrated, had a vague and dreamlike quality (Foulkes and Vogel; Rechtschaffen and Foulkes). If awakened at this point a person might feel he had been thinking or indulging in reverie. Left undisturbed, however, he will soon descend into another level of sleep.

Stage 3

The spindle bursts and somewhat irregular brain wave ryhthm begins to be interspersed with large slow waves. These occur at about one a second, and are high in amplitude. The electrical input may run as high as 300 microvolts in stage 3, as compared with the 60 microvolts of the waking alpha rhythm. Now it will take a louder noise to awaken the sleeping person or animal, perhaps a repetition of his name. His muscles are very relaxed. He breathes evenly, and his heart rate continues to slow down. His blood pressure is falling, and his temperature continues to decline. Innocuous sensory events are making almost no impression on the awareness of the sleeper, and were he among the people who do sleep with their eyes half open, he would not be seeing anything (Fuchs and Wu, 1948).

Stage 4

This stage might be called a most oblivious sleep. The muscles are very relaxed, and the person rarely moves (Jacobson et al., 1964). It is hard to awaken him with the low noise or buzzer that would have aroused him earlier. His heart rate and temperature are still declining, and his respiration is slow and even. Waken the volunteer now with a loud noise or by calling his name and he may come into focus slowly, and may feel that he was not experiencing any mental activity (Rechtschaffen et al., 1962, 1963; Kales et al., 1963). The EEG pens scratch out a continuous train of slow, high amplitude waves. The sleeper is utterly removed from the world, although his brain wave responses would indicate that every sound and the lightest touch are received in his brain. Indeed, during this synchronous, slow-wave sleep the brain shows a very large response to outside stimuli such as sounds, but the brain systems that make this stimulation into conscious sensation appear not to be working in their usual way (Allison, 1965; Hernandez-Peon, 1963; Rosner et al., 1963; Williams et al., 1962, 1964; Weitzman and Kremen, 1965). This may account for the eerie apparition, the somnambulist, who will rise from bed in this stage of sleep, negotiate a room full of furniture, look straight at people with eyes open, yet appear not to perceive them, and return to bed, usually recalling nothing of the interlude when awakened (Jacobson et al., 1965). Stage 4 appears to be one of the times when children commonly wet their beds, a time when a person is, by some criteria, most deeply asleep (Pierce et al., 1961, 1963; Scott, 1964). Although people can be trained to discriminate between sounds, to hear spoken words, to press a button during another stage of sleep, their performance during stage 4 is not nearly so frequent (Granda and Hammack, 1961; Mandell et al., 1965; Williams et al., 1963).

A normal person will spend a considerable portion of the night in this stage, especially if he has lost sleep (Agnew et al., 1964). If annoyed from outside, he will tend to drift into a lighter phase of sleep, but if annoyances prevent him from spending a certain portion of his night in stage 4, on subsequent nights he will make it up by spending substantially more time in stage 4. Although he seems hard to awaken from this phase, paradoxically he may be even harder to awaken from the first stage of sleep—if he happens to be in the throes of dreaming.

Stage 1 REM

About an hour or so after falling asleep, the

27

sleeper may begin to drift back up into the lighter phases of sleep (Dement and Kleitman, 1957). Roughly 90 minutes have passed, and the volunteer's sleep has resumed the pattern of stage 2. Now, suddenly, the pens of the EEG begin to jabber, scratching out wild oscillations. He has turned over in bed, and moved. As the oscillations die away the brain wave record shows an irregular low-voltage, rapidly changing script like that of stage 1. Now two pens that are activated by movements of the eyes make rapid darts, as if the eyes had turned to look at something. Intermittently the pens continue. The eyes move as if following a film (Aserinsky and Kleitman, 1955; Dement and Kleitman, 1957; Roffwarg et al., 1962). These rapid eye movements, known as REMs, signal a phase of vivid dreaming, a most unique state of consciousness (Dement, 1965). In this phase, it will take a relatively huge amount of noise to awaken a person—yet a very slight noise, with significance, may quickly alert him (Goodenough, 1963).

Sound a click in the sleeper's ear, and his brain wave response will not resemble that of stage 4—but shows a great resemblance to the response during waking. Although it may be hard to awaken a person at this time, in many ways his brain activity paradoxically resembles waking, and REM sleep is often called paradoxical sleep. It is believed by some investigators to be a unique state, totally different from the rest of sleep, and subserved by different brain mechanisms.

The entire body shows pronounced changes now (Snyder, 1960, 1962, 1964, 1965). Gone is the even breath and pulse. The organs that show the most striking changes in sleep are those indicating fright or anger. Everyone is familiar with the blanched skin, wide eyes, rapid heart beat and knotted stomach of fright. These changes are controlled by the closely related nerves of the autonomic nervous system, which regulates the organs of the chest and viscera, changes in the skin and eyes, with the help of hormones secreted by the adrenal glands. The autonomic system modifies its organic domain in unison, and is tuned in to the emotional state of the creature. During slow wave sleep the heart rate, respiration, and blood pressure fall to their lowest levels of the day, falling at sleep onset and continuing to drop until about an hour before awakening. During REM sleep, however, the heart rate, blood pressure, and respiration become exceedingly variable, sometimes fluctuating wildly. Usually there is a long interval of REM sleep during the latter part of the night, the time when a person's temperature has fallen to its nadir. During the REM period in the early hours of morning the activity of the autonomic system often becomes most intense, inducing what have been called "autonomic storms," which may account for the statistically frequent occurrence of heart attacks at this time, and further study of this period may make it possible to anticipate and prevent such coronaries.

Many of the physical changes that attend the REM state can be observed from watching the sleeper. At the onset the muscles of the head and chin will relax completely (Berger, 1961; Jouvet, 1963; Jacobson et al., 1964; Dement, 1965).

This is so regular that the loss of tonus in the muscle under the chin can serve to activate an alarm, signalling the onset of REM sleep. Most teeth-grinding occurs at this time (Reding et al., 1964). From infancy through adulthood, the REM period is attended by penile erections in males (Fisher et al., 1965). Rapid, jerky movements of the eyes can be seen, even in many blind people (Berger et al., 1962; Gross et al., 1965).

Most striking of all, however, is the now substantial evidence that this is a period of vivid dreaming for all humankind, and the suggestion that it is a period of consciousness in which monkeys and perhaps other animals experience vivid imagery. Awakened during REM sleep, a person will almost inevitably report mentation that differs from waking thought, dramatic, and often bizarre—generally recognized as a dream (Dement and many others). Yet, if he is awakened a few minutes after the rapid eye movements cease, when he has lapsed into another phase of sleep, the dream will have evaporated. The average individual spends a total of about 5 years of his life in such vivid dreaming, but for the most part he is amnesic, remembering very little.

The discovery of the REM phase of sleep and subsequent findings about the body and brain during this state have raised many fundamental questions about the organization and function of the central nervous system, and has stimulated a rapidly growing body of research which will be explored at greater length in later sections of this paper.

It has been said that the average adult dreams

about every 90 minutes, and that the full cycle of sleep stages spans an interval of 90–120 minutes, corresponding to a subcycle within the circadian temperature rhythm.

This generalization is somewhat misleading, although it has been widely propagated in the press, for dreaming, dreamlike experiences, fragments, images, mentation occur in all phases of sleep, although recall varies. Sleep is a succession of repeated cycles. Nevertheless, one's progression through a night does not resemble the passage of a train on a circular track, arriving at different stations at a predictable time. People of about the same age do not follow such a rigid timetable of sleep, and all humanity does not rise and fall on the waves of a single tide.

The Whole Night

A reexamination of the nightly EEG patterns of sleep has been conducted recently with 16 medical students, each of whom spent four nights in the laboratory. Only two uniform patterns emerged. The entire group showed a greater incidence of REM periods during the last third of the night, and the slow-wave sleep of stage 4 predominated during the first third of the night. Not only was there no consistent time schedule of sleep stages for the group—but individuals showed slightly different patterns on different nights. Excepting for their REM periods they did not spend more than 10 minutes at a time in any EEG phase, and throughout the night stage 2 with its spindles occurred evenly, like a transition period, a bridge (Williams, Agnew, and

31

Webb, 1964). Evidence from a number of studies suggests that each of us has a characteristic sleep pattern, an EEG script that is identifiable and individual, although we vary somewhat from night to night. So far no rules have been found for describing the succession of EEG phases that all people will pass through in a night's sleep, but more sophisticated analyses may indeed reveal an inherent order in the sequence of cycles (Zung et al., 1965; Hammack et al., 1964).

However much people differ in detail, normal people show roughly the same overall pattern. They sleep for a long interval once in 24 hours, at the time of their lowest body temperature. They spend roughly the same proportion of the night in REM sleep and stage 4, distributing them over the night in roughly the same manner.

Marked deviations from this pattern are often signs of serious disorder. Encephalitis is an extreme instance, and its sufferers may suddenly find their daily temperature cycle inverted; they will sleep by day and remain awake at night. Or they may sleep for weeks after enduring periods of exhausting insomnia. Among some encephalitis patients, unusual EEGs have been noticed in sleep, such as extraordinarily slow spindles. Epileptics commonly have seizures during certain phases of sleep, and Drs. C. Markham and R. Walter at UCLA have observed bizarre EEG sleep patterns in some patients who alternated between stages 1 and 2 and never exhibited the patterns of deeper sleep. A characteristic abnormality of many narcoleptics is that REM activity begins at the onset of sleep instead of an hour or so later;

while a tendency of some psychotic patients is to have delayed and reduced REM sleep. These deviations all speak of different disorders in the central nervous system, some of them perhaps of a metabolic nature. Normative studies, encompassing individuals of all ages, may make it possible to clearly describe the protocols of the nighttime nervous system—yielding a diagnostic by which disorders can be pinpointed. Sleep is a convenient time for study, since the body is still and there are few distractions. It is not incongruous to use sleep EEGs in diagnosing many behavioral symptoms, for sleep is not separate from waking but seems to be a part of a neurophysiological continuum that ranges from coma to the high arousal of fierce rage.

Analysis of the EEG

It must be apparent that sleep does not consist of four distinct EEG stages, but this has been a convenient taxonomy, established in the 1930's and 1940's, when electroencephalography was finding diagnostic use. As approximate categories, the EEG stages of sleep have been useful, like national boundaries, although there appear to be subdivisions within, difficult to define in a visual interpretation of the record, and beginning to show up more clearly as computer techniques are employed for analysis.

There are many problems in visual analysis of the EEG. The massiveness of the record is one. When a volunteer in a sleep laboratory first begins to stretch and regain the strength of his relaxed muscles after the night, he has left behind him a manuscript that covers almost 2,000 feet of graph paper. If he wore only 8 paired electrodes there will be 16 lines of script. Except for gross body movements which visibly slash the script with gigantic spikes, most of the changes are small and subtle—taking place continuously, sometimes within seconds. It is not always easy to determine frequency at a glance, and counting the number of waves per second is a laborious procedure. If many hundreds of nightlong records are needed to depict a normal night of sleep, it seems clear that the paper record is too enormous to analyze efficiently.

A worse problem arises when the scientist must eke detailed information from the record. If he were comparing the sleep patterns of two individuals, he might reasonably ask several questions. Is stage 4 in one person identical to stage 4 in the other? To answer this question he might want to compare similarly timed segments from each record. Are they equivalent in the coherence and stability of the rhythm? Are they alike in the relationship between brain-wave frequency and voltage? These are fairly rudimentary questions, but a single example will illustrate how monumentally difficult it has been to answer them by visual techniques. Following a hunch that the relation between frequency and voltage might be an important characteristic of certain EEG phases of sleep (the number of waves per second as related to the amplitude of each wave) one scientist examined a few minutes of the record visually. To do so, it was necessary to make photographic enlargements, so big that a relatively few seconds of record covered a wall in the laboratory. Only then could wave amplitude be measured with any accuracy, by ruler. Such a time-consuming method would be useless in a normative study, in most researches, and rapid diagnostics. Fortunately, computer techniques have made it possible to get such information in a reasonable time.

During the last 5 years there have been many developments in the analysis of the EEG data, using computers, and a good number of these have come from the pioneering work of Dr. W. R. Adey and his laboratory, not a few deriving from space research, and having such unlikely origins as the analysis of missile vibration. These, however, are the methods that are making the EEG a sensitive instrument, capable of divulging vastly more information about the workings of the mind, whether waking or asleep. In the future one will hear a great deal about averaging portions of the EEG record, of power spectra analysis, cross-spectrum analyses, phase-amplitude measures, and calculations of equivalent noise bandwidths. These techniques have already had a noticeable impact on the study of sleep (Adey, 1963).

In an increasing number of laboratories, EEGs may be monitored visually, but they are also recorded on multichanneled magnetic tape. By the proper manipulations the tape can be given to the computer, which does the dog-work of counting waves per interval, or screening for certain voltage. Each wave on the record has a certain frequency, and the EEG spectrum consists of the distribution of waves among these frequencies. The computer can be asked to do the counting, and spectral analysis will describe this distribution, showing frequency changes that might be imperceptible to the eye. Similarly, by assigning a number to each point on the wave, voltages can be handled numerically, and related to frequency by a digital computer. The emerging figures will depict the distribution of energy in the physical sense, the power spectra. Power shifts have been used to map subtle changes in attention and a progression of changes from alertness to sleep. Spectral density analyses have shown the changing distribution of energy as an individual shifts from alertness to drowsiness and sleep. During wakefulness the energy may be spread among the high frequencies—the fast waves—and as drowsiness begins there is a gradual increase of energy among the low frequency components of the brain waves. Researchers are using this method to obtain a detailed picture of energy changes in the human brain during waking performances and different phases of sleep. Because it is so sensitive to changes of attention, this technique shows great promise for future use in the diagnosis of the mentally ill.

Phase analyses describe the relative timing of trains of waves, telling which leads and which lags behind the other, and by how much. Analysis of phase shifts has proven useful in exploring the way the brain changes during learning, and may enhance our understanding of the memory process in all states of consciousness, perhaps revealing why memory of sleep is so notably poor (Adey and Walter, 1963).

Small EEG segments that look coherent and

stable to the eye have been shown to contain many variations, when analyzed by a plotting of frequency bandwidth against duration. Dr. Adey's laboratory has used this "stability diagram" to discriminate between seemingly coherent intervals, and has shown clear and unambiguous differences between phases of sleep that were once thought to be almost identical—and between wakefulness and REM sleep, whose configurations were often confused by early encephalographers.

A vast proportion of our current work on sleep depends upon the EEG, but what is an EEG? How can what is happening inside the brain be known by recording from its surface? The EEG has been roughly likened to the sound of a running motor. One can tell a great deal about a motor by its noise, comparing its sounds with performance. Still without opening it up, it is not possible to infer the precise organization or the exact contribution of any part by simply listening. So with the EEG. The inference that a pattern of brain waves taken from the scalp represents a rhythm at a site deep within—is a composite from many studies. Some of these may correlate behavior with the EEG; they may come from animals in whom deeply implanted electrodes show what happens at a subcortical locus while EEG's are obtained from the scalp. Some come from studies of normal and intact people. Others may come from patients about to undergo neurosurgery, in whom implanted electrodes and scalp electrodes give simultaneous readings during behavior and different states of consciousness (Chapman et al., 1962).

What is being recorded from the scalp? This EEG picture appears to be the waxing and waning of electrical potentials in cells of the cortex, large numbers of cells. Using microelectrodes that penetrate a single cell, it has been shown that individual neurons transmit in a rhythmic manner in discharges of pulses and pauses, and they also process information by an independent wave process. Instead of becoming neutral after it fires, the cell appears to reverse its polarity, thus oscillating between negative and positive charge. Its timing may be paced by the electrochemical constitution of its membrane, and there are thought to be several ways in which the discharge rhythm is influenced. It may be influenced, for instance, by its nonneural envelope, the glial cells. These cells are thought to modulate the excitability of nerve cells by enhancing and reducing their electrical resistance. Thus, the EEG does not reveal directly the action of individual brain cells, but indicates shifts of potential among masses of them.

When the EEG pattern is regular and synchronous, masses of cells are shifting polarity together, like a crew of oarsmen rowing together. This synchrony is characteristic of the alpha state— about 8–12 cycles per second (cps), and a number of neurophysiological studies suggest that the pacemaker for this rhythm may lie in the thalamus. Synchrony is also characteristic of deep, stage 4, sleep, and indeed was once an EEG synonym for deep sleep. The neural metronome for this cortical synchrony is not known, although it is thought to lie deep within the brain. During waking, the cortical rhythm is generally desynchronized, and animal experimentation has pointed to the reticular formation in the brain stem as an important promulgator for the signals permitting arousal. Oddly enough, however, the irregular, low voltage, rapidly changing brain waves that characterize waking are seen—in very similar form—during sleep. The pons portion of the reticular activating system prominent in waking has been shown to be important during REM sleep—that curious state of outward oblivion in which a person or animal is hard to awaken, yet shows cortical rhythms that resemble those of waking.

The puzzle is just beginning to be unravelled. What minute changes in the rhythms emanating from controlling centers, what shifts of command and organization account for these different states of consciousness and different EEG patterns? Many scientists have postulated that our states of consciousness swing in the balance between that of the dominant activating system and a hypnogenic system, a neural network that produces sleep when it is excited. These shifts occur within the core of the brain, and emanate to the cortex through an enormous and complex system of nerve fibers that connect the cortex with the deep subcortical reaches within.

In our attempts to solve the puzzle of the origins of EEG patterns, the sources of the rhythms of consciousness, we have relied heavily on animal studies, with a few exceptions. However, in the course of evolution, mammalian brains have changed in structure and distribution of functions. Recent studies have underscored the difference between lower mammals and man. One exploration suggests that the distribution of sleep phases in chimpanzees and man may be regulated by the amygdala, far forward in the temporal lobes, rather than in more basal regions. EEG rhythms, not seen in lower animals during sleep, have been spotted from the amygdala of the chimpanzee and man (Adey et al., 1963; Rhodes et al., 1965).

Human studies are therefore, important, and fortunately modern techniques have made brain probes increasingly safe and productive of relevant information. Many clues to the local residence of certain EEG configurations have come from studies of pathological symptoms, and from autopsy. Because of its variety of strange effects upon sleeping and waking patterns, encephalitis has stimulated considerable research, most notably perhaps, after the epidemic that raged through Europe after World War I. Today, however, clinical studies of patients are likely to be coordinated with laboratory experiments upon animals, and a variety of techniques are focused upon the same phenomenon. In this fashion, the behavior, the brain waves, and the possible brain centers for activity are slowly matched with surface recordings.

The process of inference and cross-correlating of many kinds of data is methodical and slow, but the results have an almost magical quality, for like reading the Bible from the head of a pin, a researcher can look at a few squiggles, lasting no more than 5 thousandths of a second, and see how a signal travels through different brain areas and something about how the brain is processing it. Whenever a sensory signal occurs, a light, sound, touch, etc., the brain reacts, and its response appears in a transient, visually indistinct pattern on the EEG. However, if the signal is repeated and the EEG response patterns are superimposed upon one another and averaged, random variations in the EEG pattern known as "noise" will fall away, leaving a clear picture. This averaging technique has permitted us to penetrate the sleeping brain through surface electrodes, because the latency, duration, amplitude, and direction of the EEG response can be measured and will yield information about the state of the brain they were taken from.

This technique has been used by Dr. Burton S. Rosner and his colleagues on normal volunteers (Rosner et al., 1963; Goff et al., 1962). A signal was repeated in waking, and throughout the stages of sleep, adding to data from other laboratories, and further elucidating the functional differences that seem to typify our many states of consciousness. Many people have shown that the brain emits a smaller response to incoming sensory stimuli during waking and dreaming than during deep sleep. Yet the deeply sleeping person does not seem to be disturbed by his breath on the pillow, sounds, or touches, despite the fact that his brain shows a large response. Perhaps his obliviousness can be explained, for sensory stimuli must be integrated and processed within the brain before they become felt. They may be received but not felt, unless they are integrated. If a brain wave response is divided for the analysis of its parts it seems that the sensory reception occurs first, but there is an ensuing pattern that is thought to represent activity at a higher station in the

41

brain. This comes very late in deep sleep, and with high amplitude. Hence sensory inflow may show a greater response from the specific sensory fibers in sleep than in waking, yet there is almost no perception, for something has changed in the integrating process. Some people believe that this shift in the mode of action occurs in the diffuse projection system and its thalamic connections between the cortex and the core, and further experiments are being designed to test this hypothesis.

Summary

While the examples cited here will be pursued more fully in other sections, they may illustrate how many levels of sleep research are converging to produce insight into the function of the brain, creating tools of great diagnostic value. The study of a night's sleep may entail, at the gross level, methodical observation. By watching a sleeping person throughout the night, for instance, there are evident physiological changes. There are clusters of muscle twitches, rapid eye movements, intervals of stillness, periods of body movement, periods of even breathing, and times of uneven breathing. These have been correlated with the scalp EEG portrait, showing that there are cyclical changes in nervous activity sweeping through the cortex. These represent changes in mentation, consciousness. Data from many sources, from deep brain studies, anatomical studies, and preoperative probes in human patients—have begun to show us how to interpret the surface EEGs to understand the organizational changes within the brain, the shifts of function and activity that appear as the striking patterns of nightly sleep. At the same time, computer techniques of EEG analysis are effectively making the EEG a far more sensitive and informative indicator of brain activity. A great number of sleep studies are clarifying the normal picture of nightly sleep. It now seems likely that the EEG of sleep may become a useful diagnostic, an instrument that can point to specific loci of disorder, suggesting something of the mechanism of an abnormality rather than simply indicating a deviation from the normal pattern. New methods of analyzing EEG data, supported by a variety of data, may therefore be able to take us deep within the brain so that we can see, with surface electrodes, activity in regions that in past years required neurosurgery for exploration.

Chapter III.
Sleep Deprivation

Man, often in laudable arrogance accompanied by blinding ignorance, has always attempted to exceed the limits of his own physical nature. The obvious needs—hunger, thirst, respiration—have been accorded respect as essentials to survival. The very word "starvation" has its roots in the Old English word "sterve" (to die) ; and the connection between lack of food and death has been plain throughout the world's history. Sleep has been a different issue without the status of a drive, although sleep deprivation has long been used as torture. Before we can answer why we sleep, or how much sleep we need, modern civilization appears to be racing to eliminate sleep. This is a heady prospect, for, if successful, it would add about 20 productive years to the lifetime of the average man. Nevertheless the question remains: must we sleep? Is sleep an integral part of our organic rhythms, our metabolism? One useful procedure for exploring body needs is to deprive— take away sleep and see what happens. In the 1950's, following World War II, a large number of volunteers underwent periods of sleep starvation in laboratories where they were measured for physiological and chemical changes, their ability to perform tasks, and where their psychological changes were under continuous scrutiny. Anyone who seriously thinks of eliminating or drastically reducing his sleep should examine this literature.

We have all been exposed to anecdotal "proofs" that certain people can manage well without sleep—long vigils of sleepless performance by medical interns, the so-called charrette or 3-day drafting binge of the architect, a spate of remarkable incidents retold after World War II, famous "wakathons" endured by disc jockeys, and last year an 11-day stint of sleeplessness by a 17-year-old high school student in San Diego. Despite the lack of sleep the architects drafted winning plans, the interns treated the sick, the disc jockeys gave their usual performances, soldiers won battles—and after a night's sleep, we are told, they were fresh as ever. Studies performed at the Walter Reed Army Institute of Research, largely by Dr. Harold L. Williams and his associates, have told a discouraging story about a person's performance during prolonged wakefulness. Several of the famous wakathons were, at least in part, studied by scientists, and these too offer some disheartening information about the psychological effects of going without sleep for long periods, as well as raising questions about aftereffects. One disc jockey, with a record of some mental instability, went 7 days without sleep, endured persistent symptoms even after rest, and ended in a mental hospital, although a stable young high school student apparently recovered from a much longer stint with no noticeable aftereffects.

The mental symptoms of prolonged sleeplessness seem to occur slowly, in a somewhat predictable fashion, mounting, as the time goes on, sometimes into very dramatic proportions. At Walter Reed and elsewhere one of the most consistent observations was the progressive unevenness of mental functioning, lapses in attention, growing fatigue, weariness, and a tendency to withdraw from the outside world. People began to make fewer and fewer unnecessary movements, and showed some confusion between their own thoughts and external events. Certain bodily sensations began to develop. A tightness around the head gave the impression that a hat was being worn. Many complained that their eyes burned or itched and their vision was blurred, after 30–60 hours of sleeplessness people had difficulty with depth perception. Small objects seemed to dart out of place, and chairs changed apparent size. Commonly, lights seemed to wear a halo of fog. Even the floor seemed to undulate. By 90 hours, some people developed vivid hallucinations. One volunteer, for instance, called for help in washing the cobwebs from his face and hands. Brief dreams would intrude and become confused with reality, and people found their time sense distorted. These symptoms, along with changes of mood and deterioration in performance, were disturbing enough, and were recorded in detail in the definitive Walter Reed studies that did not extend the sleep starvation beyond 98 hours (Williams, Lubin, and Goodnow). If the sleep-loss is protracted beyond 100 or 200 hours, however, it appears that the symptoms intensify and begin to resemble psychosis. The fifth day has seemed to be a turning point in a number of cases observed (West et al., 1962).

Temporary Psychosis

In January, 1959, the largely unaware public saw before its very eyes the kind of temporary psychosis that can be induced with sleep starvation. Under the supervision of doctors and scientists, Peter Tripp, a 32-year-old disc jockey, undertook to stay awake for 200 hours in a Times Square booth for the benefit of the March of Dimes. Throughout this marathon of over 8 days, Tripp was given medical and neurological examinations, tests of performance, psychological tests, and was closely attended by Drs. Harold L. Williams, Ardie Lubin, Louis Jolyon West, Harold Wolff, William C. Dement, and others. Although his experience was undoubtedly worsened by the tension of publicity and public conditions, some of the ordeals of Peter Tripp may indicate the kind of mental symptoms that can beleaguer the severely sleep starved.

Almost from the first, the desire to sleep was so strong that Tripp was fighting to keep himself awake. After little more than 2 days and 2 nights he began to have visual illusions; for example, he reported finding cobwebs in his shoes. By about 100 hours the simple daily tests that required only minimal mental agility and attention were a torture for him. He was having trouble remembering things, and his visual illusions were perturbing: he saw the tweed suit of one of the

47

scientists as a suit of furry worms. After 120 hours he went across the street to a room in the Hotel Astor, where he periodically washed and changed clothes. He opened a bureau drawer and dashed out into the hall for help. The drawer, as he had seen it, was ablaze. Perhaps in an effort to explain this and other visions to himself he decided that the doctors had set the illusory fire, deliberately, to test him and frighten him. About this time he developed a habit of staring at the wall clock in the Times Square booth. As he later explained, the face of the clock bore the face of an actor friend, and he had begun to wonder whether he were Peter Tripp, or the friend whose face he saw in the clock. The daily tests were almost unendurable for Tripp and those who were studying him. "He looked liked a blind animal trying to feel his way through a maze." A simple algebraic formula that he had earlier solved with ease now required such superhuman effort that Tripp broke down, frightened at his inability to solve the problem, fighting to perform. Scientists saw the spectacle of a suave New York radio entertainer trying vainly to find his way through the alphabet.

By 170 hours the agony had become almost unbearable to watch. At times Tripp was no longer sure he was himself, and frequently tried to gain proof of his identity. Although he behaved as if he were awake, his brain wave patterns resembled those of sleep. In his psychotic delusions he was convinced that the doctors were in a conspiracy against him to send him to jail. On the last morning of his wakathon, Tripp was examined by Dr.

Harold Wolff of Cornell. The late Dr. Wolff had a somewhat archaic manner of dress, and to Tripp he must have appeared funebrial. Tripp undressed, as requested, and lay down on the table for medical examination, but as he gazed up at the doctor he came to the gruesome decision that the man was actually an undertaker, about to bury him alive. With this grim insight, Tripp leapt for the door, and tore into the Astor hall with several doctors in pursuit. At the end of the 200 sleepless hours, nightmare hallucination and reality had merged, and he felt he was the victim of a sadistic conspiracy among the doctors.

With some persuasion, Tripp managed to make a final appearance in the glass-windowed booth in Times Square, and after his broadcast he went to sleep for 13 hours. Although the record of his ordeal covers hundreds of pages, the few instances cited here may give some indication of the extreme distortions, mental agonies, and delusions he suffered, especially during his last 100 hours of sleeplessness. When he awakened after his first long sleep the terrors, hallucinations, and mental deterioration had vanished. He no longer inhabited an unstable visual world where objects appeared to change size, where a doctor's tie would jump out of place, and where it was a superhuman effort to solve a simple problem or remember an anecdote. In 13 hours of sleep the nightmare existence had been left behind, although for 3 months afterward Tripp suffered a mild depression. Quite aside from the quick apparent recovery from extreme symptoms, there had been two extremely striking patterns throughout the ordeal, periodicities that suggested that Tripp's times of strength and moments of worst symptoms followed some inner cycles. Throughout the ordeal Tripp had been able to organize and perform his daily broadcast. Temperature readings showed that he was at his peak at the broadcast time, the point of his highest daily temperature. His bursts of hallucination and strange behaviors, on the other hand, seemed to occur in 90–120 minute intervals, at times when he might normally have been dreaming. At the time this periodicity suggested a possible physiological link between the mechanisms of dreaming, psychotic symptoms, and hallucination. In retrospect some of the observers feel that the most impressive changes were those that followed the diurnal cycle.

The Role of Age

Six years ago, when Peter Tripp began his marathon of wakefulness, he was 32 years old. Last year, a 17-year-old high school student set out to break the record, and in the quiet atmosphere of his home, without the help of coffee or other stimulants, he stayed awake for 264 hours. Drs. L. C. Johnson, W. C. Dement, and J. J. Ross were on hand for observation and medical examination. Here there was quite a contrast to Tripp's wakathon.

Randy Gardner did, indeed, show progressive changes with sleep loss. By the fourth day he became irritable, suffered lapses of memory and difficulty in concentrating. He saw fog around street lights, felt the band of pressure of an illusory hat, and imagined a street sign to be a person. By

50

the ninth day he seemed to think in a fragmented manner and often did not finish sentences, sometimes experiencing transient reveries. His eyes bothered him, and he became unsmiling and expressionless. At one point, about the fourth day, he had imagined himself a great Negro football player. He did not, however, show extreme symptoms, and at the end of 11 days, he slept for over 14 hours, and rebounded into a healthy and cheerful mood. During the last few days of his vigil, however, he had shown definite neurological changes. His vision was blurred, and his right eye was making involuntary sidewise movements. Whether his eyes were open or closed, his alpha rhythm was markedly reduced, and he showed waves characteristic of sleep. The usual alpha wave enhancement to external stimuli was no longer present. Physiological measures indicated that during deprivation the basal autonomic pattern was one of activation, but also that there was less responsiveness to outside stimuli. For example, during deprivation there was marked vasoconstriction. Randy's heart rate rose above normal. His skin temperature and electrical skin resistance were very low. As time went on these indices, which usually show changes in response to external events, became less and less responsive. When Randy finally went to sleep, however, all of these measures showed responses to external stimuli, save only the galvanic skin response. On the first night of sleep after his vigil, his EEG showed a different pattern than on successive nights. It contained a concentration of slow wave (stage 4) and stage 1 REM. Ten days after the vigil, Randy

51

was clear of all symptoms except for slight difficulty with memory and involuntary eye movements (nystagmus) (Johnson, et al., 1965; Ross 1964).

These two very different individual reactions illustrate several important aspects of sleep loss that have been corroborated in other studies. Randy Gardner, by psychiatric measures, withstood his long vigil with greater ease and less effect than any of the people who had so far been recorded beyond 120 hours of sleep loss. His own home and the attendance of his own family physician provided surroundings that were less exacerbating than those of Peter Tripp or others, even on shorter vigils in the laboratory. He took no stimulants. But perhaps equally if not more important, were his youth and his general stability.

A person's reaction to prolonged wakefulness would appear to be congruent with his personality patterns and what might loosely be called stability. From interviews and psychiatric tests of 74 army volunteers in Walter Reed studies, researchers found they could predict reasonably well which individual would find the experience most difficult and would report hallucinatory events (Morris and Singer, 1961). Some years ago, at McGill University, six chronic schizophrenic patients were kept awake for 100 hours. As sleep loss continued these patients began to show acute symptoms that had not been seen for several years among them, auditory hallucinations (Koranyi and Lehman, 1960). The extent of a person's suffering under protracted sleep loss would seem to depend upon what we term mental health, and the six publicly recorded wakathons that have been undergone in recent years seem to highlight the point that symptoms occur sooner, and with greater intensity, in unstable individuals. There is also some evidence, however, that age may be an important factor.

Randy Gardner, who set the record for a sleepless vigil, was the youngest person to attempt this stint. Further evidence that young creatures may withstand sleep loss for longer periods than older ones has come from the laboratory of Wilse B. Webb at the University of Florida. The finding was serendipitous because it arose from a rat study that was not designed to explore this point. Originally, the experimenters had designed a continuously rotating mesh wheel, two-thirds submerged in water, in order to keep rats alert without causing muscular exhaustion so that they would fall asleep instantly when placed in a recording cage. Rats avoid cold water, and the wheel moved slowly enough so that they would not fall in if they kept awake and moved very slightly. Because the original wheel was small, it could not carry a fully grown animal, and so the first experimental animals were very young, about 63 days old.

The experimenters expected the creatures to last atop the wheel for several days, but were surprised to see them maintain position day after day. Some lasted 27 days before they fell. This feat of wakefulness raised some interesting questions. How had the young rats managed to stay awake, continuously moving for 27 days? The experimenters speculated from other data that these flexible young animals had not yet formed rigid sleep patterns and were able to sneak short naps of a few seconds. The only way to corroborate this

53

hunch was to obtain continuous EEG readings while they were astride the water wheel, and see if characteristic brain waves of sleep appeared in the record. It was technically impossible to obtain EEGs from rats 63 days old, for there was then no way of implanting electrodes into the small and delicate brain. The repeated experiment had to be conducted with older rats, whose brains could be implanted with tiny electrodes. The older rats were about 200 days old.

When these adults were placed upon the water wheel, however, they had no staying power. They fell off in 3 to 4 days. The experimenters immediately began testing rats of intermediate ages on the wheel. The animal's age was directly correlated with the number of days he would last upon the wheel (Webb, 1962). In order to gain some insight into this differential staying power, the experimenters developed techniques for implanting young animals. They have recently found that the young animals manage to spend a surprising amount of their time asleep. By running to one edge of the turning wheel they can then ride with it, catching a nap of 10–15 seconds before they must quickly move to avoid falling. By this maneuver, the experimenters have estimated the animals may spend a third of their time on the wheel asleep. They are evidently very tired by the time they leave the wheel; nevertheless, the young rats manage to spend long periods atop the wheel in this fashion, whereas the older rats cannot. It does seem, at present, that age bears some relation to the ability to withstand sleep loss, and this capacity may be associated with the ability to snatch brief naps, although the reasons may be multiple and related to metabolism, especially in rodents, and muscular vitality as well as "habits" of the nervous system.

Physiological Changes

Although next to nothing is known about the psychological changes that may be occurring in animals as they are deprived of sleep some changes have been observed (Webb, 1962; Kleitman, 1963). It is largely from animals that we have learned about the damages that sleep loss may induce in brain tissue. From histological studies of animals experimenters infer that there may be certain changes in human brain tissue during sleep loss. How these may vary with age is not known. The published case histories suggest that many of them must be reversible, and the recent study of Randy Gardner suggests that youth may be an advantage in recovering from sleep loss. It should be repeated, however, that subtle aftereffects, perhaps not noticeable to Randy or to a casual onlooker, persisted for 10 days, and perhaps months after the vigil. Aftereffects have been difficult to measure and evaluate in human beings, and the question of tissue damage is unanswered at present. Studies of sleep loss have been relatively few and recent, and the question of prolonged, perhaps even indefinite, aftereffects remains an unsettled one. There is no way of telling whether the severity of aftereffects may be in proportion to the pathological symptoms experienced during sleep starvation.

Perhaps it is worth citing a few of the animal experiments that have shed a little light on this question. As early as 1894 M. de Manaceine demonstrated that cerebral hemorrhages took place in puppies when they were kept awake to the point of death. Tissue damage in the cortex and frontal lobes was reported by Daddi in adult dogs kept awake, fatally, from 9–17 days. Nathaniel Kleitman kept puppies awake for 4–6 days, and many died. They, too, had suffered cerebral hemorrhages, and the number of red blood cells had dropped to about half of the normal count. Other changes in neural tissue were observed in sleep-deprived dogs by Legendre and Pieron, and these were shown to be reversible if the animals were allowed to sleep. Sleep-deprived rabbits showed cell changes in the spinal cord and brain stem, and so, depending upon the species, it might seem that some of the clinical signs observed during sleep deprivation come from cell changes in the cerebral cortex and brain stem. In some of the many animal experiments a single period of sleep restored the animal to normal after a moderate deprivation (Kleitman, 1963). However, nobody can be sure that a long period of sleeplessness or the habit of skimping on sleep for months or years will leave no permanent ill traces. At present we have no way of determining what changes may leave a subtle, lifelong effect, perhaps even a chain reaction, enhancing disease, perhaps shortening the life span. Animal and human studies have indicated some of the physiological changes that occur when sleep is prevented for long intervals.

Abnormal amounts of nitrogen and potassium have been found in the blood and urine of sleep-deprived animals. Glandular and hormonal changes have been observed as well, and it is interesting that experimenters report irritability and belligerence in sleep-starved animals, like that of sleep-starved people.

Several studies suggest that the body metabolism suffers difficulty during prolonged wakefulness, and these suggest one of the ways in which normal sleep may be regulated. The body appears to be governed by internal clocks, intermeshed systems of biochemical change that we call metabolism. One of the cycles we have come to recognize is a diurnal rhythm of rising and falling temperature in man. In the Walter Reed studies oral temperatures were taken during a 98-hour period of sleep deprivation, and it was clear that the diurnal rhythm remained. Indeed, people felt most sleepy and tired at the time when their temperatures were lowest. During the progressive sleep loss, in addition, the overall body temperature declined somewhat. Perhaps this was an indication of a declining metabolism, a progressive inability to produce energy (Williams, Lubin and Goodnow).

Energy Metabolism

The awake person, however quiet, is placing demands upon his nervous system and his musculature far in excess of the activities of sleep, thus draining the energy reserves of his body. A biochemical study of two sleep-starved volunteers—one wakeful for 5 days, the other for 10 days—suggests that biochemical mobilization of energy changes considerably after 4 or 5 days without

57

sleep. This may account for the pathological symptons and delirium that have been observed after 5 days of sleep loss (Luby et al., 1960, 1961). The body's transformation of food energy into a form useful to muscles, nerves, and all cell activities depends upon a single chemical. It is adenosine triphosphate, known as ATP, which seems to be the catalyst for energy release in all living matter. Every cell, at any given time, has a certain proportion of this nucleotide with its three phosphoric acids. As food substances are transformed into cellular energy, ATP breaks down from a triphosphate into ADP—adenosine diphosphate. By a process known as phosphorylation ADP and adenylic acid combine to make more ATP, which is stored with creatine as reserve energy. However, during prolonged activity the stored supply is used up, and new ATP must be created. At about 4 days of sleep deprivation, the production of the three critical energy substances of the body appears to run down. This seems to be the evidence from studies of six individuals at the Lafayette Clinic (Luby et al.). At first, energy production seemed to increase by an emergency process of synthesizing chemicals not usually utilized. But after the fourth day, the emergency metabolism seemed exhausted. This was the time when the subjects showed most striking changes in personality and performance, experiencing the weird phenomena associated with delirium. The fact that sleep returned the energy systems to normal and restored the individuals to normal behavior suggests that sleep may be essential to the body's system of energy production, that it is integral to metabolic functioning.

These biochemical studies instigated new interest in the relation between sleep loss and mechanisms of mental illness. Clinicians have long observed that sleep disorders, particularly insomnia, often precede a first attack of mental illness or an acute episode in the mentally ill. During sleep starvation, even the functioning adult can be swept into the unreal world of a transitory mental illness. Although we do not know what specific biochemical changes activate particular neural mechanisms to cause visions, distortions, and hallucinations, we have now seen that the severe symptoms appear at a time when the body's energy metabolism has utilized emergency means to produce energy and may not be producing a normal ratio of transmitter chemicals. The approximately 5-day turning point is a point of extremely low ebb and fatigue. Studies report many changes long before that, inattention, changes in mood, visual and tactile illusions. Even after 36-48 hours' sleep loss has produced noticeable effects.

Another possible link in the chain of metabolic events has only recently been discovered by scientists who have been exploring the body's reaction to stress. During sleep loss, as the Lafayette group has indicated, the energy metabolism first acts on an emergency basis as if sleep loss were a stressor like insulin. After stresses such as fright or frustration, changes in hormonal output and noradrenalin can be detected in the blood: corticosteroids that are secreted in extra quantities by the pituitary adrenal glands. There has been considerable speculation about what part of the brain tells the pituitary to shift into emergency production. The suggestion of another biochemical link in the metabolic and mental changes of sleep loss had its roots in a discovery of a brain region in humans that may take part in issuing the command for the extra production of stress hormones. During the early 1960's, Dr. Arnold Mandell and a team at UCLA found an elevation of corticosteroids in epileptic patients who had undergone presurgical exploration and had received gentle electrical stimulation in the amygdala, a portion of the brain that is frequently involved in temporal lobe disease. The amygdala, far forward in the brain, seemed to play some part in the neural command system by which the adrenal-pituitary glands are induced to pour hormones and stimulants into the blood during crisis. This finding led to a further exploration of the chemistry of stress. Using normal volunteers, under mild stress, they injected ACTH, which acts as a hormonal stress and is indeed one of the pituitary hormones. ACTH stimulated adrenal production. Moreover, when the blood and urine were put to chemical analysis, a new and previously unknown substance had appeared. This chemical was repeatedly produced by artificial stress. It belonged to a family, the indoles, related in structure to serotonin and LSD–25. Subsequent studies were to demonstrate that this indole—signal of stress— might appear in the blood even before there was any elevation of stress hormones, possibly preceding the emergency action of the pituitary-adrenal glands in some instances, and possibly signifying a separate biochemical system operating in stress (Mandell et al., 1963).

Studies of normal people under food or sleep deprivation followed. When volunteers went without food for 2 days there was almost no significant rise in stress hormones, but the indole appeared. After only 48 hours of sleep deprivation the indole was detectable, although stress hormones increased after 24 hours. Should this stress-responsive indole have psychotomimetic effects like LSD, and increase during progressive sleep loss, one might expect that it plays a role in the behavorial changes observed (Mandell, et al., in press). This new evidence of biochemical change, during early sleep loss, again suggests a link between sleep, metabolic processes, and symptoms of mental illness. Because it is so vague, the word stress is usually avoided in describing sleep loss and other events. Looked at as a chemical signal of stress, in some colloquial sense, however, the appearance of this indole suggests that sleep loss, like other stressing events, causes biochemical reactions that may be clues to the etiology of mental illness.

The biochemical traces of prolonged sleeplessness have been explored only recently in human beings. The weakening impact of sleep loss—the fact that it produces confusion, disorientation, and even delusion—must have been known throughout history. The standard trick of the villainous has been to deny captives sleep (West, 1957). This is still a tool of the police in extorting confessions, and an inherent part of some military interrogations. Because protracted sleep loss can produce

61

psychotic symptoms that are erased by a period of sleep, it has been said to break the will without leaving scars, providing one of the cheapest, most traceless and humiliating forms of torture. Apparently, it has been one of the more successful techniques of Communist interrogators, and the subjective agonies of the transition to exhausted unreality are well known as described by Arthur Koestler in "Darkness at Noon." Presumably sleep-loss psychosis occurred among some of the U.S. fliers in the Korean conflict: people who signed confessions of germ warfare and could not, later, account for their own behavior. The leeched and hollow-eyed suspicious stare that has characterized the faces of many sleep-deprived volunteers has been seen by everybody in the trial photographs of the tragic Cardinal Mindszenty, who presumably suffered continued sleep loss and interrogation before he publicly confessed to being a spy. The fact that protracted sleep loss can induce effects like those of a temporary psychosis—disorientation of time, place, person, and identity; confusion, inattention, visual illusions, hallucination, and delusional thinking—has provided a tool for exploring mental illness experimentally from many sides. During the last 10 years many new tools have been added to the scientist's armamentarium, so that behavior, EEG events, physiological changes, and metabolic changes can be correlated.

Psychological Changes

The psychological changes observed in sleep-starved people surely prompt questions about the

62

relation between fatigue and moral behavior. No studies have been designed specifically to probe this point, although, indeed, sleep starvation appears to produce some behaviors that might be considered a weakening of moral character. Long before the appearance of gross psychotic symptoms, for instance, an individual experiences sheer fatigue and will start to economize on muscular and intellectual effort to shift from one activity to another when left to his own devices and indulge in listless and transitory social interactions. (Murray et al., 1958, 1959). As one laboratory study suggested, a person may begin to take the easy way out, choosing the strategy that demands the least of him. Although this indication of laziness says nothing about moral decisions under fatigue, it suggests that the study of sleep loss may have many social implications. The world might, indeed, be different if everyone got 9 hours sleep, and if key decisionmakers were not among the least rested members of society. Such speculations must go unexplored for the moment, but there is a large body of information of great social relevance, in the thorough behavioral studies conducted in the laboratory of Harold L. Williams at Walter Reed.

Sleep Loss and Performance

These studies begin to answer some very practical questions about man's ability to perform while deprived of sleep, at the same time exploring some of our most basic questions—why we sleep, and what happens when we don't. Under the recurrent exigencies of combat or work deadlines people are not ordinarily deprived of sleep for

10 days at a stretch. But 3, even 4 day vigils have occurred in battle, among seamen, and professionals. At Walter Reed, during 1956 and 1957, a first group of volunteers was kept awake for 3 days (72 hours) while a second group attempted 4 days of unremitting wakefulness. The point of the studies was not to push the men to the limit and examine psychological abnormalities, but to examine thoroughly their abiltiy to perform certain tasks. The volunteers, all of them young army men, lived out their experimental period in a well-equipped hospital ward, attended by nurses and corpsmen, and were subjected to the same battery of tests at the same hour each day. The staff maintained a 24-hour watch, keeping drowsy volunteers awake; food, coffee, and recreational facilities were amply provided at all times. This was an unharrassing setting and permitted companionship and some esprit. As the sleep loss progressed the men reported increasing irritation with their eyes and vision, a few suffering illusions such as the apparent vision of steam rising from the floor, cobwebs, or hair in milk. Intrusive thoughts, or fantasies, the hatband illusion, and time distortion occurred. From outside one might have said that their mental processes were slowing down. They would lose their train of thought, make mistakes in speech, sometimes meandering off into a fantasy. As they filled the long hours between tests, the young men quickly shifted from reading and playing complicated games to desultory conversation, avoiding intellectual effort (Williams, Lubin and Goodnow).

Most people realize that it is advisable to avoid

driving a car, flying a plane, or performing other manipulations that require split-second reactions if they have been deprived of sleep. Safety manuals sometimes say that reaction time slows down with fatigue. After about 30 hours, as the Walter Reed subjects showed, reaction time became very uneven. A man might take three times longer than normal, on the average, to respond to a signal, but at times he would react quite as rapidly as he had before sleep loss. Sometimes, however, he would take a very long time to react. He was not simply and steadily slowing down like an unwound clock as sleep loss went on, but he seemed to be missing signals altogether, growing progressively more uneven on reaction time tasks. The net effect might have looked like a radical slowing of response time. In fact, the volunteers were progressively experiencing more and more lapses of attention in which they utterly failed to get the signal.

Reaction time tests generally require a subject to press a button or perform a manipulation whenever a certain signal occurs, but the subject has no control over the pacing of the signals. As the Walter Reed team began to distinguish between the tasks that suffered most during sleep loss and those that seemed resistant, it became clear that sleep-starved people did far better when they were allowed to set the pace themselves. They could, for instance, maintain accuracy in solving problems. Allowed to take as much time as they wanted, the volunteers could add pairs of numbers accurately (Loveland and Williams). If pressed to add rapidly, yet accurately, the subjects managed to do arithmetic correctly by finishing fewer problems. They could not sustain accuracy and speed. A person who could set his own pace performed far better than he did when paced by somebody else.

When playing a communications game in which one volunteer issued orders and another executed them, the person issuing the orders made fewer errors than the subject following them. As sleep loss progressed, however, both made more errors, and by 70 hours into their vigil they doubled the number of errors they had made in a rested state (Schein, 1957).

A wealth of eminently practical information emerged from the Walter Reed studies, and although this was not their most important contribution, it is worth reciting some of the results. In the initial studies, monotony seemed to worsen the performance of the sleep-starved volunteers, yet upon further testing it appeared that monotonous jobs such as tracking an uncertain signal generated more errors than highly redundant yet tedious tasks. Accuracy of scanning could be maintained by sacrificing speed. Performance could be improved if the person received feedback, telling him the results of his moves. Incentive also improved performance. So did a challenging and competitive task. R. T. Wilkinson, of Cambridge, England, tested a game that simulates a naval battle, and found that sleep-starved subjects performed well despite fatigue. On the other hand, progressive sleep loss took its toll when a person had to cope rapidly with added increments of information; for instance, a volunteer could rapidly sort cards into 4 categories under progressive sleep loss, but could not speedily sort them into 10 categories (Wilkinson, 1964). With progressive sleep loss the volunteers became less efficient at optional tasks. When playing against the standard slot machine, for instance, the normally rested volunteer tried to vary his moves so as to "beat" the machine. However, early in his vigil the same man would adopt a rigid and predictable strategy, no longer trying to keep in mind past plays that might reveal the machine's program. It was as if he no longer cared and were alternating his choices in the manner that cost the least mental effort.

Performance was not the same at all times of day and night, but tended to show the most deterioration in the early morning hours during the low point of the daily temperature cycle, improving during the next day, afternoon and evening. This daily temperature cycle became slightly exaggerated during sleep loss, and the volunteers felt most fatigued during their periods of lowest temperature. Symptoms, lapses of attention, intrusive thoughts, illusions, skin sensations, and dreamlike experiences also clustered roughly between 5 and 7 a.m., when the person would ordinarily have been sleeping. The volunteers also showed a different reaction to background noise when they were sleep-starved (Wilkinson, 1963). Normally, a rested person will fare worse at a vigilance task when there is a hissing noise in the background, but this hissing seemed to improve the performance of the sleep-starved.

At first glance, there is something very strange and inconsistent about the behavior of sleep-starved people as it has been described in the literature. They can read yet find it difficult to follow simple orders. Peter Tripp managed to organize and conduct his daily broadcast, yet found it hard to perform simple tests. Volunteers might react swiftly to a signal in one instance, yet utterly miss a signal the next time. A crucial test of sustained attention was used at Walter Reed and highlighted the nature of this seemingly strange combination of incapacity and capacity among the sleep-starved. This was the Continuous Performance Test designed by Rosvold and Mirsky of NIH (Mirsky and Kornetsky, 1964). The subject merely had to press a lever whenever a particular sequence of letters appeared amongst a continuous parade of letters across a screen, or when a sequence of sounds was heard among a continuous train of sound; or when a particular vibration occurred among others. As sleep loss progressed the subjects made more and more errors of omission, whether the signal was visual, auditory, or tactile. These lapses were a key to his progressively uneven performance on other tests—for he was missing things.

These lapses in attention had been observed before, and studied by Bjerner and Liberson. The brain wave recordings of Walter Reed volunteers soon indicated what had been happening. A subject, wearing electrodes, could perform a tactile or auditory vigilance task while reclining with his eyes closed. The EEG record taken at the time of his lapses showed that the characteristic alpha rhythm of wakefulness had slowed down. For brief moments, perhaps 2–3 seconds, bursts of slow waves appeared, resembling those of sleep. The person seemed to have experienced a brief seizure of sleep, which has long been referred to as a microsleep (Liberson, 1945). Thus a person, setting his own pace, might slowly but accurately solve a problem or read a paragraph—but if the text were read to him, a microsleep might cause him to miss a word or phrase and thereby to misunderstand. He might miss a number and compute incorrectly. On a scanning task, he might miss a signal on the radar screen—and from an error of omission, be led into an error of judgment and action. Microsleeps become more frequent as sleep loss continues, interfering with a person's reception of outside information.

These transient lapses have not been blamed for peculiar psychological effects, and a humorous biographical incident in the writings of Mark Twain suggests that microsleeps might be blamed for a host of superstitions and reported apparitions. In his manuscript "Mental Telegraphy," Twain recalls watching a stranger approach his house, and then vanish. Twain, convinced he had seen a bona fide apparition, hurried to the spot, and then inside. He found the man sitting in the inside hall, having rung and been ushered in by the servant. Not having seen this, Twain concluded that he had been asleep or totally unconscious for about 60 seconds, while the man rang and entered the house. If the man had gone elsewhere in the house, instead of waiting in the front hall where Twain could see him, Twain confessed. ". . . thirty yoke of oxen could not have pulled the belief out of me that I was one of the favored ones of earth, and had seen a vision—while wide awake."

Sleeping on one's feet is no myth. Where long vigils are essential—as perhaps in an industrial mission, a space trip, or a military operation—it seems clear that self-paced tasks, group tasks with inherent competition, and high incentive tasks are to be preferred over sentry duties, surveillance, or monitoring for sleep-starved personnel. Increasingly frequent microsleeps, the influence of the temperature cycle, and evidence for a rhythmic occurrence of dreamlike intrusion in 90-120 minute intervals provide some new guidelines by which we can now design the tasks and work schedules of people on long and potentially sleepless duties. We are only just beginning to realize that sleep requires the same kind of attention we normally give to the logistics of food, sanitation, and other essentials.

Summary

The study of sleep starvation to date has underscored a number of factors worth restating. Progressively, as sleeplessness is prolonged, a person suffers sensory disorders—illusions of visual and tactile sensation that may eventually develop into hallucination. Lapses of attention, microsleep intervals become frequent. There is a tendency to withdraw from activity, to become disoriented in time, and place, and person. The extent of the effects are influenced by many environmental factors, but psychological symptoms may be related in their intensity to the mental stability of the individual. Age seems to be a significant factor, and there is some evidence that it is easier for the young to withstand and recover from long vigils.

As reflected in the brain wave patterns, a characteristic effect of sleep loss is the slowing of the waking alpha rhythm. Reduced responsiveness to sensory stimuli occurs on autonomic measures, although heart rate, for example, has been found to be somewhat accelerated. Stress hormones in the blood show an elevation very early in sleep loss, and signs of biochemical changes occur within 48 hours. The energy metabolism of the body is altered, showing a severe decline at about 120 hours and coinciding with the onset of psychotic symptoms.

Although a single night of sleep appears to erase most of the symptoms, there is no saying at this point what subtle traces may persist, nor how these may be related to the age and usual mental state of the sleep-starved individual. The effects of chronic sleep loss are almost unknown, and we do not now know how a habit of reduced sleep may influence waking performance or lifelong health. EEG studies of volunteers on schedules of restricted sleep have shown that there is one immediate effect, an alteration in the person's usual EEG pattern of sleep (Sampson, 1965; Webb and Agnew, 1965). Eight young men in a University of Florida experiment cut their sleep to 3 hours a night for 8 days. During these nights their sleep was not simply a miniature, a compression of their usual nightly pattern, for they spent about as much time as usual in deep stage 4 sleep, at the expense of other sleep stages (Webb and Agnew, 1965). As this study progresses, it may reveal whether a habit of reducing sleep produces behavioral effects, and whether there are cumulative disadvantages.

Surely the behavioral studies of sleep loss performed at Walter Reed suggest that, however subtle, the effects can be socially and individually undesirable. Among the least mentioned is the intense desire to sleep in people who must, for whatever reason, stay awake for long periods.

Must we sleep for long periods, or could we train ourselves to nap? Do we need a certain amount of sleep for sanity and health, or could we reduce sleep radically? These questions have not been answered by experiments in sleep deprivation, although some of the studies have been undertaken in order to determine changes in metabolism or other biochemical events that may reveal how sleep is normally controlled. For a start they have shown that sleep loss, and the continuing activity of wakefulness, incur biochemical changes and metabolic alterations, and these may be related to the coincident pathology—the tortured and psychotic behavior that has characterized most of the severely sleep-starved adults observed so far. Sleep loss induces a variety of abnormal symptoms in otherwise normal people, and it is interesting to note that sleep disorders, notably insomnia, are commonly precursors to acute episodes in the mentally ill.

Chapter IV.
Sleep Disorders

The very symbol of peace and well-being is the silence of a darkened town asleep; it is a lonely figure in a lit window who may be in trouble. The healthy, the fortunate, succumb to sleep casually, accepting it as naturally as breath, enjoying a respite from worry, grief or pain, and awaken refreshed. Without this nightly suspension, the wealthy are poor and the poor destitute. The inability to sleep, or stay awake, or a disorder in the recurrent cycle of sleep can become a torment and disrupt a life with appalling speed. Sleep disorders can alter a person's mood and behavior to a degree that is often ignored, and mood, activity, and environment play their part in altering sleep. Sleep disorders are a concomitant of many mental illnesses, and it has been said that anyone who visited the wards of a mental institution at night before the wide use of tranquilizers stepped into a living hell.

The most common sleep disorders are those that accompany a physical or mental disease, but there are others, characterized by inappropriate sleep, such as narcolepsy, encephalitis, and certain forms of epilepsy. Studies of these various sleep abnormalities have enlightened some of our speculations about the normal mechanisms of sleep, and have underscored the fact that sleep is not an isolated event, but part of a rhythm that involves the entire person, his body chemistry, his mental outlook, his behavior, his emotions, and his environment.

Insomnia

Insomnia, whether real or imaginary, has become so widespread that it helps keep the drug companies in business, especially in large cities where tranquilizers and sedatives are consumed by the trainload. Most adults have had difficulty falling asleep in times of trouble or worry, and during the fever or pain of an illness. Elderly people and depressed patients often find that they awaken long before they wish, in the dawn or predawn hours. In its many forms, insomnia probably constitutes one of mankind's most subtle tortures, but many people apparently think they are tormented with insomnia at times when they are actually asleep.

To date few studies of insomnia have been conducted in the sleep laboratory. One of these, performed in the 1940's by Dr. W. T. Liberson, showed that insomniac patients alternated between periods when their brainwaves showed the large waves of sleep, and periods giving patterns of alertness. During the brief episode of sleep the patients would snore, but later deny having slept, presumably because of the rapid alternation with alertness. Nurses, having heard the snores, would insist that the patient had been sleeping soundly.

74

During the late 1950's, Dr. Arthur Shapiro, at New York's Downstate Medical Center, recorded the nightlong EEGs of several professed insomniacs. Several volunteers complained that they had not slept very much all night, but their brainwaves indicated that they must have been asleep, dreaming they were awake. Since that time a number of laboratories have seen instances of "wakefulness" during which people were actually sleeping.

Perhaps the most startling confusion of sleep and wakefulness took place in the University of Chicago Sleep Laboratory in late 1963 when Dr. Allan Rechtschaffen and his associates were tracking the process of falling asleep. In this pilot study, subjects went to sleep with their eyelids taped half-open. When their EEGs indicated the first stages of sleep, a lighted object was held before them. A few seconds later they were awakened and asked about their thoughts. In a sequence of many such awakenings one subject never saw the illuminated comb or cup before his eyes, but persistently asserted that he had been alert and wide awake—thinking. His thoughts were fragmentary images, often resembling brief dreams.

An interesting and detailed study of the drowsy state has been performed by Drs. W. T. and Cathryn W. Liberson of the Stritch School of Medicine, Hines, Ill. They, too, have found the distinct EEG patterns of drowsiness in people who denied being drowsy and claimed they were just thinking. The eyes began to roll slowly during the first onset of drowsiness, increasing for some seconds, and then diminishing and disappearing as sleep spindles appeared on the EEG. As the drowsy patterns invaded the EEG, even subjectively alert subjects showed a sudden shift in attention from present reality to vague thoughts of the kind everyone experiences in the midst of daily activity. The Libersons have suggested that it might be a biological necessity to blur the environment occasionally, entering an intermediate state between vigilance and dreaming (Liberson and Liberson, 1965).

Other volunteers in the laboratory of Dr. Donald Goodenough have asserted they were awake and thinking when aroused from a dream period following a long interval of sleep. They have reported—as thoughts—long and bizarre dream narratives, and their subjective confusion of sleep and waking may suggest that they sleep "lightly," for they have explained that they could control their dreamlike thoughts in the manner of daydreams and were aware of sounds in the room, such as the noise of an air conditioner.

Imaginary insomnia is no joke to the person who exacerbates his problem by growing tense over his supposed inability to sleep; and its possible causes are of great interest. A study performed by Lawrence Monroe, which is summarized in a later chapter, indicates some of the striking physiological and EEG differences among individuals, characterizing what has loosely been called good and poor sleep. These seem to be correlated with personality factors and health. According to the data collected so far, it does seem that people vary considerably in the "depth" of their sleep, and that some people may retain greater contact with the outside world and subjectively feel awake at times when they think they are in control of their dreamlike experiences and thoughts.

People hospitalized for the treatment of depressive illnesses, have shown generally abnormal sleep patterns as judged by EEG recordings (Gresham et al., 1965). Indeed, EEG records of sleep have been seen, so abnormal as to be hard to interpret by the usual EEG guidelines, and these were the sleep records of persons with severe classic depressions (Hawkins et al., 1965).

An early study of depressed patients with subjective insomnia indicated that these people took longer to fall asleep than their normal counterparts, and moreover, spent twice as much time in a light phase of sleep from which people usually report dreaming or thinking (Diaz-Guerrero et al., 1946). Nurses in hospitals have observed patients who lay motionless in apparent sleep, yet claimed they were awake. These people seem to sleep in a higher than normal state of physiological and neural arousal, and it has been suggested that the fault may lie within an arousal or vigilance system of the brain, partly located in the brain stem reticular formation near the base of the skull. Why do these people complain? Why do many of them feel unrested? Does light sleep prevent the body from metabolizing energy in sufficient quantities? The answers to these questions are unknown at present, but it is reasonable to assume that many of these people suffering imaginary insomnia are not exaggerating when they complain of insufficient rest.

A Neural Pacemaker

Subjective insomnia may, in some cases, reflect a subtle sleep disorder that has nothing to do with insomnia, strictly speaking, but may instead reflect an unstable shifting of the nightly sleep pattern. Instances of instability, a restless shifting of the EEG phases of sleep, were noted in depressed patients who thought themselves wakeful (Diaz-Guerrero et al.). The possible source for this apparently abnormal cycle was recently under-scored by UCLA sleep studies of epileptic patients. A number of epileptic patients or people with intolerable motor disorders have undergone pre-operative examination by means of electrodes deeply implanted in the brain. Among them, two patients showed a bizarre EEG during sleep. They oscillated between the lightest stages of sleep, at 10-minute intervals, never showing the brain wave patterns of deep, stage 4 sleep. Both of these patients had severe damage in the tem-poral lobes and showed seizures that were gener-ated in the hippocampus and amygdala. This observation is of great interest, for the amygdala is known to be associated with emotion, with inte-grative processes, perhaps with short-term memory and pituitary stress mobilization. Now there is evidence that the amygdala may regulate the pro-portions of sleep that a person spends in the sev-eral EEG phases.

Adey and his associates at the Space Biology Laboratory of UCLA have found that a chim-panzee's sleep closely resembles man's. In studies of implanted chimpanzees, the investigators noted spindling patterns from the amygdala during REM sleep, an unusual pattern that has since been seen in implanted patients, but not in other animals. In recent experiments with monkeys, moreover, the experimenters disconnected the amygdala and found that the animals now spent a different proportion of their sleep in the several EEG stages. If the amygdala plays some role in apportioning the EEG states of sleep in men, investigators may be able to track a number of sleep disorders to their neural locus. The new evidence suggests that while graded sleep stages in lower animals may be governed in deep subcortical regions of the brain, man and infrahuman primates have evolved a shift of these controls so that the site of the mechanisms governing sleep have moved into the forward regions of the brain near the cortex. The amygdala, a small bulge of tissue at the front end of each temporal lobe, has long been associated with emotion. If this region participates in the pacing of the stages of sleep, we may begin to uncover the neurophysiological link between emotional difficulties and sleep disturbances.

Sleep Disorder and Mental Illness

Because sleep disorders and mental illnesses almost inevitably occur in concert, sleep disorders have become a cue for clinicians in discriminating between similar forms of mental illness. If typed by sleep symptoms, depressed patients, for instance, appear to fall into three distinct categories. Some people oversleep in what we have often dubbed escapism. Others become too anxious and agitated to fall asleep at night. Still others fall asleep easily but awaken too early in the morning.

Drugs also discriminate between types of illness. In treating depressed patients who, by clinical classification, are anxious rather than hostile, certain drugs are far more effective. One kind of drug that has particularly benefitted some somnolent and anxious patients is a chemical that interferes with a complex chemical chain that destroys norepinephrine in the brain—the monoamine oxidase inhibitor. One such psychic energizer, iproniazid, has enabled several depressed patients to function well for over a year on 3–4 hours of sleep, possibly by promoting more efficient brain metabolism and reducing the need for sleep (Bailey, et al., 1959; Kline, 1961). The differing sleep patterns and drug responses of depressed people suggest that we have lumped several different ailments under a single name. Further study of the normal chemistry and neurophysiology of sleep may, indeed, help us to ascertain the physical components of the moods and behavior of these various patients.

Surely sleeplessness, or complaints of restless sleep, have become warning signals for the physician. Many mental illnesses and suicide attempts are heralded by troubled sleep and a visit to the doctor for sleeping pills. The connection between mental illness and disorderd sleep is plain in any mental institution at night when, despite tranquilizers and sedatives, the hours of darkness become filled with restlessness, nocturnal terror, agony of mind. It is only in recent years, the last three or four, that sleep studies have been launched among the institutionalized in the hope of understanding, predicting, and controlling symptoms that are correlated with unusual sleep patterns.

A survey of several hundred hospitalized psychiatric patients has indicated that about 70 percent of them experienced sleep disturbances before they were admitted for treatment. They either fell asleep with difficulty and awakened during the night, or had a pattern of awakening very early with the feeling that they had not slept soundly; two patterns typical of depression. Many of them resorted to medical help because of their insomnia, and were administered tranquilizers or sedatives. Interestingly enough, there were more suicide attempts among the patients receiving sedatives or tranquilizers, than among those who were given antidepressants. In addition, patients who said that they had been dreaming less, or that they had stopped dreaming, also showed a tendency to attempt suicide (Detre, et al., 1965).

At St. Elizabeths Hospital, the Federal hospital of about 8,000 patients in Washington, D.C., a team of NIH doctors has undertaken a long-term study of the sleep of psychotics and elderly people suffering chronic brain syndromes (Feinberg, Koresko, Gottlieb, Wender). Here, volunteer patients live for several weeks in a special ward where they adjust to the laboratory, get acquainted with the staff, and are under continual observation. A very simple procedure has enabled the doctors to follow progressive sleep disturbance and predict behavioral deterioration. A laboratory attendant makes a half hourly check on each patient all night,

81

noting whether the person sleeps, is awake, or is in an indeterminate state. The resulting chart has produced a striking pattern. The number of awakenings during the night, or the amount of insomnia, is easy to measure and does predict deterioration. Sleep deprivation experiments have demonstrated that lack of sleep, alone, can produce deterioration in behavior—even symptoms like those of psychosis—and that sleeplessness is accompanied by biochemical changes in the body. It is not surprising that sleep loss, even relatively mild, should exacerbate the symptoms of psychotic patients.

In schizophrenic patients, the sleep pattern may enable an important diagnostic distinction. Some patients do not suffer sleep disorder before a breakdown but sleep like babies. This group, unlike the larger group of schizophrenics, is little helped by tranquilizers. Possibly the symptoms suffered by these people have roots in different neural mechanisms. In the great majority of schizophrenics, for whom tranquilizers offer real relief from symptoms, acute episodes are usually preceded by increasing insomnia, and it has been postulated that these patients suffer from excessive activity in the arousal system of the brain.

In an EEG study of 22 patients, the St. Elizabeths' team has observed a great restlessness in the sleep of schizophrenics that is characterized by turnings and twistings of the body. Hallucinating schizophrenics have also shown unusual amounts of eye-movement activity during their dream periods, and while this may have little to do with visual imagery, it again suggests a high state of excitation, possibly within reticular activating mechanisms. The elderly people who show signs of disorientation and confusion and who cannot remember recent events have also been distinguished by different sleep patterns. Some show a great deal of REM activity, but others show abnormally little. Two volunteers, whose sleep was particularly light, awakened during dreams in the laboratory, ripped the electrodes from their heads and were urgent to leave the hospital for "an appointment." These two people showed a great deal of eye-movement activity during REM sleep, suggesting hyperarousal. Further studies, correlating sleep patterns, behavioral symptoms, and responses to drugs may help to define what is now a rather vague designation of arousal (Feinberg et al., 1964; Koresko et al., 1963).

Common Disorders

Insomnia, restless sleep, or distortions of the sleep rhythm as depicted by EEG fluctuations are undoubtedly the most common and often the most serious complaints that come under the heading of disordered sleep. Many other sleep behaviors, however, come to the attention of the family physician. Some of these are nuisances, such as snoring and sleeptalking. A well-known annoyance, bedwetting, is relatively common among preadolescent children, occurring in about 5–15 percent of them, according to one estimate. Adult enuresis is surprisingly frequent, occurring in perhaps 2 percent of the population. The Army, an admittedly selected population, has found bedwetting in about one man in a hundred. Until recently it was generally assumed that wetting occurred during dreams, perhaps as the result of dreams, but current nightlong EEG studies demonstrate that this is not so.

Drs. Chester Pierce and Roy Whitman, working at the Cincinnati Medical School found that enuretic boys of 5-9 and adults 17-21 generally skipped the first REM cycles, possibly because they were unaccustomed to sleeping in the laboratory. Their wetting occurred in the deepest stage of sleep, stage 4. Drs. David R. Hawkins, George Thrasher, and Jimmy Scott at the University of North Carolina, have shown that wetting occurs in several stages of sleep—generally just before a dream episode, and least frequently in REM periods, a finding confirmed by Broughton and Gastaut (Gastaut and Broughton, 1964; Hawkins et al., 1965). Children in the studies had generally shown gross body movements prior to wetting, and when awakened reported no dreaming, although apparently dreaming often followed. If many sleep disturbances seem to signify arousal, enuresis by contrast seems to occur in heavy sleepers, children who are often hard to awaken. Physiological records taken in the Cincinnati studies show that the enuretic child frequently has other disorders, some showing EEG abnormalities, some sleepwalking, many enduring urinary complaints such as pressure, overly frequent need to urinate, even pain. These supposedly healthy children also had an unusually high nitrogen content in their urine (Pierce et al., 1961, 1963; Saint-Laurent et al., 1963). A drug that effectively lightens sleep, imipramine, has looked promising in getting children to stop their bedwetting, but it also produces an irritated mood.

Teeth-grinding (bruxism) and head-banging, by contrast, appear to happen mostly during dreaming sleep. Teeth-grinding seems to be a result of normal contractions occurring in the masseter muscles during REM sleep but is particularly forceful among tense persons (Reding et al., 1964).

Somnambulism

Sleeptalking and snoring are annoying to others but relatively harmless, while bruxism often causes dental problems. One of the most eerie and fascinating of sleep behaviors—sleepwalking—is not always innocuous to the performer. Somnambulists have been known to perform remarkable feats—to stride across narrow walls, pick their way through furniture, and negotiate around obstacles without harm. Some, however, have jumped out of windows, like the young woman, recently described in a newspaper report, who was found in the street with broken legs. As she explained to the police, she had a vivid dream of eloping with her fiancé and had merely opened the window and stepped onto the ladder, which unfortunately existed only in her dream. Many of these weird occurrences have been associated with traumatic incidents, like the nightly struggle of one French marine who rebattled a fire and mutiny at sea, colliding with chairs and tables so violently that he wounded himself visibly in sleep. And yet, upon awakening he felt he had slept calmly. Because of its repeated association with vivid dreams in the reports following the event, somnambulism has been thought to be an enactment of dreams. People reasonably expected that it would occur during the REM phase of sleep associated with vivid dreaming, a period when the scalp EEGs bear resemblance to the waking brain wave pattern, but until recently the evidence remained anecdotal, composed mainly of happenstance observations or reports to clinicians (Riser, 1962, and many others).

An EEG study of somnambulism, performed last year by a team of researchers at UCLA yielded the startling and provocative information that walking did not occur in REM dream stages—but in the deep, slow-wave sleep of stages 3 and 4, a period not currently thought to be associated with intense dreams. This initial study was conducted with 4 volunteers who had been selected from 25 sleepwalkers, children, and adults. A special cable permitted the subject to leave his laboratory bedroom, while wearing his garland of electrodes connected to the EEG machine, while EEGs were continuously recorded. Each slept in the laboratory for 5 nights, and during this time the investigators studied 41 somnambulistic incidents. In each instance of walking or getting out of bed, the activity began in stage 3 or 4, and usually the subject did not remember having moved.

As the subjects moved around, the synchronous, large waves of stage 4 diminished in amplitude, progressing toward a lighter stage of sleep, and another interesting brain wave configuration was observed. During the actual sleepwalking, a regular wave, resembling the alpha rhythm of relaxed wakefulness, entered the brain wave pattern. Although normally the alpha rhythm vanishes when a person opens his eyes, this rhythm did not vanish when the sleepwalker opened his eyes.

The open eyes of the subjects lent a strange quality to their appearance, for they walked around furniture and people as if they could see—yet showing little sign of recognition or appearing indifferent. Their faces were blank, their feet shuffling, and they did not seem to perceive the investigators although they looked at them. One 9-year-old boy, whose brain waves were being recorded by biotelemetry, apparently oblivious to the presence of the scientists, wandered into the monitoring room and, 30 feet to the end of the laboratory, entered a kitchen, retreated and entered another bedroom, and finally returned to bed. Ten minutes later, because one of his electrodes had developed a loose connection, one of the investigators awakened him in order to repair it. The child remembered nothing.

This study and one French study give a first glimpse of the somnambulist in action. His brain waves more closely resemble those of deep sleep than those of the waking state. However, they are different. This may point to another state of vigilance apart from waking or sleep, a state in which there is usually reduced awareness of the environment, but in which complex and even violent acts requiring interaction with the environment may be performed (Jacobson et al., 1965).

Evoked Potentials

How could a person see—take in visual and other sensory information—at a lowered level of vigilance and without remembering? Why during stage 4 sleep? Quite a number of neurophysiological studies have offered data that may explain this apparent paradox. One method of determining how the brain responds to a signal during each of the stages of sleep is to sound a click in the ear of the sleeping animal or person, flash a light, or deliver a very gentle electric shock throughout sleep. By performing the stimulation repeatedly, and by superimposing the subsequent brain wave records using an averaging technique, it is possible to gain a clear picture of the characteristic brain wave pattern that follows. This evoked potential can tell something about what parts of the brain are responding, how rapidly they respond, how sizable the response is, and how responses to any particular stimulus compare in waking and the stages of sleep. Brain wave responses to stimulation, obtained from animals and from normal people in waking and sleep, have shown that the heaviest censoring of sensory stimulation must occur during waking and REM sleep. In other words, the signals coming from specific sensory channels produce less of a response in the EEG in waking and during dreaming than in deep sleep.

There are indeed many differences too ramified for summary here. However, it would seem that the waking and REM dreaming brain maintain a focus of attention by prohibiting most of the chaos of sensory signals from entering significantly into the brain. Oddly enough, as many investigators have demonstrated, this censorship seems to be least strict during stage 4 sleep. If the pathways from the sensory nerves accept stimulation to a greater degree in stage 4, one might wonder why the sleeping individual is not disturbed by the pressure of bedclothes, or his breath on the pillow, or the sounds in the room. In colloquial terms, the explanation may be that stimulation does not become sensation—it is not experienced—until it has been processed and integrated by the brain. Studies of evoked potentials strongly suggest that these integrative functions are not operating in their usual way during stage 4 sleep. This evidence has been seen in several species of animals and in humans in studies conducted by a number of scientists (Burton S. Rosner, Jose Segundo, Raul Hernandez-Peon, and others).

In attempting to offer an anatomical hypothesis to explain the EEG responses, two investigators have phrased it differently. Dr. Hernandez-Peon of Mexico City postulates the existence of neurons, within or near the arousal system, that are essential to conscious experience. If these brain cells are inactive when the arousal system becomes inhibited during sleep, the brain might receive sensory signals yet never generate awareness. Dr. Burton S. Rosner, at the University of Pennsylvania, does not explicitly postuate "conscious experience neurons." However, he feels that the diminished amplitude of the later portions of the EEG response may mean that there is a functional change in the brain regions believed critical for consciousness—the association area and diffuse projection system of fibers from the core of the brain that finally transmit sensory information to the cortex.

Thus the sleepwalker may indeed receive a bombardment of sensory information, yet not "experience" anything. Although any speculation on the neural organization underlying this strange phenomenon is quite tentative, it does seem that stage 4 sleep may permit automatic yet complex behavior—involving certain receptor and effector systems—without the usual involvement of that mysterious component that makes a responsive brain also conscious.

Modern research tools and a variety of researches should help us to further penetrate the perplexing phenomena of somnambulism and to understand why it is so often associated with vivid dreaming—although studies so far have indicated that intense dreaming does not usually occur, or is not recalled from stage 4 sleep. The fact that sleepwalking is frequently observed among enuretics, in whom urinary problems are common, and who show unusual urine nitrogen content, and sometimes slight EEG abnormalities, may suggest a biochemical factor.

We are just on the threshold of understanding the metabolism and the neurophysiology of sleep. Indeed, we still know little about three very conspicuous diseases associated with sleep—encephalitis, narcolepsy, and epilepsy.

Encephalitis

In parts of the world where sleeping sickness is common, a resistless drowsiness is a frightening omen. Attacks of somnolence, lasting days or even weeks, may come from many causes, among them brain tumors, lesions, damages from malaria, chicken pox, German measles, syphilis, and other high-fever diseases. The most dreaded sleeping sickness of them all, however, is encephalitis, which is caused by a virus. Although it appears in many forms, it generally begins with fever, delirium, sometimes to be followed by periods of agitation and insomnia, then stupor and coma. The virus raged through Europe during World War I, freqently taking its grip after a weakening siege of influenza. It inspired considerable medical research, and Von Economo and others sought in autopsies the site of the damage within the brain.

As the data accumulated from many analyses of brain tissue, it became clear that the ravages of the virus were not restricted to a particular small spot in the brain. Lesions, or what might be called neural scar tissue from the death of brain cells, were found in the hypothalamus, that portion of brain just above the palate in man, which governs appetite, body temperature, heart rate, and emotion. Depending upon the location in the hypothalamus of brain cell damage, there could be many different effects; and lesions were also found in many other portions of the brain. Thus, subsequent studies began to explain the array of preposterous effects that encephalitis had wreaked upon its victims. In some instances the victims of the disease were known to sleep as long as 5 years. Thus encephalitis, especially in an epidemic, called attention to the role of the brain in causing sleep or wakefulness.

One symptom was particularly revealing. In the aftermath of fever, especially among children, there was often a shifting or even a total inversion

91

of the diurnal sleep cycle, so that the patient suddenly began sleeping by day and remaining awake throughout the night. This sudden shift of sleep and wakefulness in the track of a brain-damaging fever emphatically suggested that there was more than convenient habit to the sleep cycle of man. Surely the cycle, however it was developed by whatever training, had some residence in brain mechanisms, perhaps a brain clock that would turn sleep on and off, so to speak. With his observations of hypothalamic lesions, Von Economo, during World War I, postulated that the brain must contain a sleep regulating center, and that the hypothalamus contained one area that induced wakefulness, while another produced sleep. Thus the epidemic of encephalitis, with all its frightful abnormalities, inspired theories about the region of the brain stem or brain that must participate in the normal regulation of sleep. It was a striking example of the way in which abnormality of behavior may help the scientist to uncover the normal process of behavior. Although the early theories were inadequate, they generated what is now intensive neurophysiological study of sleep regulation in the brain (Kleitman, 1963).

Narcolepsy

Encephalitis is well known by name at least to the public, for it is a fairly common disease in many parts of Asia, and outbreaks in Europe and the United States have generated a sizable legend and literature. Most people, on the other hand, have never heard of narcolepsy. Although this curious ailment had the status of an extremely rare illness until recently, it may not be rare at all, for many people endure its symptoms without having a name to call them. Narcolepsy is mainly characterized by a tendency to fall asleep easily and at inappropriate moments. Before their problems were diagnosed, a number of narcoleptics have fallen asleep at the wheel of a car and crashed into a building or tree. A more frightening symptom of many narcoleptics is an overwhelming, swoonlike reaction to intense emotion. Violent anger or laughter literally makes them weak with emotion, and they may lose all muscle tension, falling to the floor and sometimes into a brief sleep that resembles a blackout. This cataplexy afflicts about 60 percent of the narcoleptics. Sleep paralysis is another disturbing symptom; narcoleptics have reported awakening but being unable to move for some minutes.

People with these seemingly sinister symptoms have gone to doctors, claiming they were epileptic, or even insane. Others, prone to napping, have deprecated themselves for laziness. A great number of narcoleptics have sought help from optometrists, ophthalmologists, and oculists, believing they needed glasses because they suffered from an inability to focus their eyes (Keefe et al., 1960). Actually this double vision stemmed from narcoleptic drowsiness. There is no way of knowing how many Americans suffer from narcolepsy, nor how many industrial or auto accidents are caused by sleep attacks. The ailment may, indeed, occur in very mild form so that some people would be relatively untouched by its symptoms. Drs. D. Daly and R. E. Yoss of the Mayo Clinic have studied narcoleptics of every degree of symptom and feel that narcolepsy occurs in many degrees of severity (Daly and Yoss; Yoss and Daly; Ganada; Gastaut and Roth).

A totally new understanding of narcolepsy has been generated by the collaborative studies of Drs. Allan Rechtschaffen, William C. Dement, and George Gulevich, one which should erase the medieval aura of fear about the syndrome. Following a hunch that the symptoms were related to the REM stage of sleep, the dream period, a series of EEG studies were undertaken. One early study showed that a narcoleptic can hold a conversation, discriminate between sounds, show other signs of being wide awake, and yet have the brain wave patterns of someone deeply asleep. A narcoleptic, wide awake, has skin conductance like that of the normal person asleep. An EEG survey of nine narcoleptics and nine normal controls quickly showed one difference in the sleeping patterns. A normal adult, according to hundreds of EEG studies, will sleep for about 90 minutes before entering a REM period. The narcoleptic will, on the other hand, begin a REM dream immediately after he falls asleep.

Nobody knows how narcolepsy is caused, although statistics about the syndrome in family groups suggests a genetic propensity. Some doctors have supposed that a brain disease is the origin, and that this disease causes an adult to regress to the polyphasic sleep pattern of the infant, in which sleep occurs in 50-minute cycles. The current studies of Dement and Rechtschaffen have, in any event, demonstrated that the narcoleptic's bizarre symptoms are merely the symptoms of normal sleep, but very ill-timed. It is not that narcoleptics need more sleep than normal people, but the phenomena of sleep—of which most of us remain unconscious—intrude into waking life. Waking hallucinations, cataplexy, and sleep paralysis are exaggerations of the events that normally occur in the REM stage of sleep. Cataplexy, for instance, is not a blackout. However, if the normal person, standing on the street corner, were suddenly to lose muscle tone as he does in REM sleep, he would fall limply to the sidewalk. If he were to fall asleep at the same time, with such swiftness, he might think he had fainted.

Recent studies of narcoleptic sleep attacks were performed on volunteers at Stanford University. One indication that the ailment is not so rare as once assumed was the response of narcoleptics to an advertisement in a San Francisco paper. A call for volunteers drew a large number of replies. Screening the volunteers was simple. Could the person tell a funny joke or spank his children without suffering a cataplectic fit? Did he suffer from sleepiness? Because laughter or anger seems to trigger cataplexy, most narcoleptics learn to avoid these emotional situations and divert their attention from the events that might endanger them. Although the symptoms are outstanding, five of the cataplectic volunteers in the Palo Alto studies had never had medical attention. At present it appears that two-thirds of the narcoleptics suffer cataplexy, but that about one-third do not.

The fact that there are many cataplectic people walking around without medical help is astonishing in itself, but it is even more astonishing in the light of the new EEG and physiological data. The attack can occur like lightning. One volunteer, a woman, had been outfitted in scalp and other electrodes, prior to EEG, eye movement, heart, and respiration measurements. She sat in a chair in the recording room and was instructed not to fall asleep until the investigator had gone into the adjacent control room. However, as he closed the door a second later, she was asleep. He awakened her and dashed to the electroencephalograph machine in the next room. By that time she was already dreaming, showing the familiar brain wave and eye-movement patterns of REM sleep. The instantaneous fall from wakefulness into REM sleep is a rare occurrence. It can happen after prolonged dream deprivation, or withdrawal from amphetamine drugs, but the normal person does not experience sleep in this way (Rechtschaffen et al., 1963; Dement et al., 1964).

In studies of narcolepsy at Stanford University and the University of Chicago, narcoleptics were observed plunging instantaneously into dreams. Normal volunteers took about 50 minutes of sleep before they showed signs of REM sleep, if they did at all, during daytime naps. It is not surprising that the narcoleptic has a very different subjective experience of sleep. The normal adult slowly relaxes, going through a long transition before he loses muscle tone in his face and neck as the REM period begins. The narcoleptic, on the other hand, feels weak when he is sleepy, and many report strange sensations in the muscles. The sleep paralysis they may experience probably involves the lack of muscle tone accompanying REM sleep—but in the awakening narcoleptic remaining muscle tension may be delayed by quite a few seconds (Dement et al., 1964; Rechtschaffen et al., 1963).

One peculiar aspect of narcolespy is its periodicity. Frequently the narcoleptic will suffer attacks at intervals of 4 to 6 hours. This suggests an as yet unknown metabolic cycle. Possibly the body generates a chemical during wakefulness that is used up during REM sleep, and the narcoleptic either overproduces this metabolite, or does not use it up in nightly sleep. A series of animal experiments at Stanford University Medical School may reveal whether the REM state is triggered by a neurochemical that is consumed during dreaming (Henry et al., 1965).

The psychological quirks and neuroses of narcoleptics are difficult to assess. Surely the symptoms place an incredible strain upon a person's life and self-control. A person who is overcome by a resistless sleep attack in the midst of making love, or who drops to the street if he listens to a funny joke and laughs, might be expected to develop some unusual behavior in reaction. However, the fact that emotion can trigger the sleep attack has intrigued people who have tried to understand its etiology. A survey of the literature indicates that many narcoleptics suffered their first attack after a trauma that occurred in early adolescence. Many of these were children of about 13 to whom a death in the family caused sudden and intense emotional upset. This may be precisely the kind of emotional jolt that Richter postulated when he predicted that trauma might cause the normally out-of-phase

97

metabolic cycles to come into phase—producing strange symptoms in a periodic fashion.

Although we are still a long way from being able to trace the concatenation of metabolic events that may be involved, studies of the brain mechanisms and brain regions that participate in sleep suggest two areas that may be affected. Extensive work by M. Jouvet and others at Lyon has shown that the pons, a region of the brain stem that is phylogenetically archaic, plays a large role in generating the characteristic REM sleep that is found in animals and man. This might be one locus of narcoleptic seizures. Other possible loci may lie in the temporal lobes, in the hippocampus and amygdala, far forward in the brain. These frontal areas may act as a clearinghouse for memory and emotional information, and there has been some recent evidence that the amygdala may help to regulate the EEG phases of sleep. A wealth of data linking emotion and sleep has suggested to R. Hernandez-Peon that narcoleptic paroxysms may originate in the amygdala—an hypothesis soon to be tested.

Although we may not know the exact chain of biochemical events, and while we cannot yet pinpoint the brain cells that activate narcoleptic attacks, it is obvious that the sleep research of the last 5 years has been applied in an unprecedented way—to the benefit of every person who suffers this malady. Findings from the many studies—which are the content of this report—have been focused upon this strange syndrome in order to illuminate its nature. It must come as a relief to physicians and patients alike to realize that the symptoms are those of sleep and dreaming. Elements of the familiar always help to remove the dread of a bizarre mystery, removing some of the psychological burden. Moreover, there are now some guidelines for a regime of medication to minimize the symptoms.

Sleep loss appears to enhance narcoleptic attacks, and, indeed, narcoleptics appear to be restless sleepers. However, most of them take dexedrine in order to stay awake, and this alone may change their sleep pattern. Among other effects, dexedrine reduces the amount of REM sleep (Rechtschaffen and Maron, 1964). Pierce and his associates Miss Olivia Nixon, Drs. J. L. Mathis, and B. K. Lester have observed that several narcoleptics had less than the normal amount of REM sleep. It is interesting that a couple of them brought bags of sandwiches to the laboratory to eat late at night. A tendency to overeat has been noticed in volunteers who deliberately underwent almost complete dream loss for several nights, and suggests an interaction of appetite mechanisms in the brain with sleep. Unfortunately, because dexedrine has a hangover effect, many narcoleptics are continually raising their dose. The result may be that they are further depriving themselves of REM sleep at night and compensating with REM attacks during the day. Clearly, in the treatment of this syndrome, the patient needs a drug to keep him awake by day, but he needs a sedative at night that does not reduce REM sleep. A combination of the tranquilizer, Thorazine, and dexedrine has been tried with good results. If, instead of taking dexedrine by day, the patient could take a drug at night to enhance his REM sleep, his daytime attacks might be decreased or even eradicated. So Drs. Dement, Gulevich, and Rechtschaffen have hypothesized. During the past several years, for many reasons, there has been a search for dream-enhancing drugs, but this research is just beginning and no such drug is yet available.

The data from sleep research, enabling the recent studies of narcolepsy, have already provided the physician with invaluable tools. For diagnosis, a simple battery of tests—including EEGs of sleep onset—will indicate narcolepsy and distinguish between the cataplectic and noncataplectic person. One of the revealing tests is absurdly simple: can the patient tell a funny joke, or openly enjoy a joke related by the doctor? A regimen to prevent sleep loss and further loss of REM sleep can be prescribed, and the doctor can reassure his patient that the untoward "spells" are, indeed, just misplaced sleep. Perhaps publicity will help to take some of the psychological onus from narcolepsy and enable people with symptoms, however mild, to seek relief.

Epilepsy

A widespread publicity campaign has been undertaken to remove the onus from another disease associated with sleep mechanisms—epilepsy. In the popular conception this ailment has been imbued with mysterious, visionary overtones, and the epileptic fit is perceived in Dostoevskian force as a grand mal seizure, beginning with an aura, and ending in violent convulsions, with the person foaming at the mouth and finally entering coma. Actually, like narcolepsy, epilepsy is a syndrome of many forms and degrees, moderately rare in grand mal proportions, although not uncommon in less severe manifestations. In Los Angeles County alone, 60,000 to 80,000 people suffer one or another of its symptoms. Generally, these are not "fits," but brief episodes of blankness or automatic behavior—smacking of lips or fumbling with clothing. Epileptic seizures are often mild enough to escape medical notice, sometimes passing as lapses in attention or daydreaming.

The link between epilepsy and sleep is just beginning to be explored. Each form of epilepsy appears to induce seizures that cluster at a particular time in the individual's diurnal cycle. Indeed, the time of seizures may prove to be a defining characteristic of the particular kind of epilepsy. Most common are seizures during sleep, and waking attacks are often followed by sleep. Like the narcoleptic, the epileptic is vulnerable to sleep loss and is warned to avoid exhaustion. Some epileptics are triggered by emotion, and, like the cataplectic patient, will be catapulted into a seizure by a hearty laugh. Psychomotor epileptics, whose seizures emanate from the temporal lobes, do not go into moments of unconsciousness, but live through episodes that resemble waking dreams which they do not remember. Because certain seizures occur only during sleep or drowsiness, EEGs have been used in diagnosis for about 25 years. Until 1958, however, patients never slept more than an hour or two in the laboratory, and moreover, the electroencephalographers usually interpreted the REM stage as a period of wakefulness on those few occasions when they saw one.

101

Today, when sleep study is warranted, nightlong EEG records are taken and interpreted according to recent findings on the normal patterns of nightly sleep.

One of the first indications that sleep might be a state of high brain activity, signs that the brain did not "go to sleep," came from epileptic seizures during sleep. Many decades ago, Dr. J. Hughlings Jackson, the great 19th century neurologist, suggested that sleep must be an active brain state, after noticing that seizures often occurred as a person was falling asleep. Anybody who pays some attention as he drifts off to sleep will notice occasional muscle twitches, sometimes startling body jerks. They are very minor convulsions, generally called myoclonus. They are brought about by a hyperactive state that impels certain muscles to contract. Myoclonic spasms are hardly the same as serious convulsions, but they are related. A study of the behavior of single brain cells, especially in regions that transmit impulses to the muscle system, has begun to explain how these and other seizures may be generated in the brain. Although this work is far removed from the clinic and the epileptic himself, a brief description may suggest what the nature of a seizure might be in its most atomic form—the discharge pattern of nerve cells within the brain.

Single Brain Cell Studies

Using cats and monkeys as experimental subjects, Dr. Edward Evarts and colleagues at NIH have placed microelectrodes into various brain cells in different regions of the brain, taking EEG recordings from each cell individually. What is the difference between the cell's activity in sleep and in alertness? Until recently people guessed that cells were simply more sluggish, that they fired less often during sleep—but this is not the picture offered by the cells. Some cells, for example, located in the visual cortex, would fire more often and respond more rapidly to flashes of light in the animal's eyes if he were asleep in the REM state, than if he were awake. On the other hand, there were certain cells that became more active when the animal awakened. A sampling of many diverse cells showed what might be called a division of labor, some firing more continuously and rapidly in waking, others firing more often and rapidly in sleep. But the pattern was not so simple.

Evarts and his associates turned to the study of monkeys. They implanted their virtually invisible microelectrode tips into neurons of the pyramidal system. The pyramidal tract descends to the spinal cord at the base of the brain stem, and this system relays outgoing messages from the cortex to the motor system—translating the desire to move a foot into the command that moves a foot. Here, in the many studies of their survey, they saw that cells followed different patterns of firing during the different EEG stages of sleep and waking. One cell might fire in a regular, continuous pattern during waking, but fluctuate wildly during REM sleep. Many cells elsewhere in the brain have shown a random discharge pattern during waking, but have fired in clusters or bursts during sleep, interspersed with intervals of silence. Indeed, on closer scrutiny, it seemed clear that the waking rhythm of certain pyramidal cells was not random. Rather, it appeared that when the animal was awake these cells were inhibited to some extent, but when the animal slept this prevailing damper seemed to be removed. Now, uncontrolled, the cells might discharge in large bursts. This is the kind of discharge that causes seizures and shows up on the scalp EEG as a great spike formation. Further exploration of the nature of the inhibiting mechanism that prevents great bursts of cell firing now continues at several levels. Although the single brain cell is the atom of consciousness, many clues into the nature of epilepsy must come from molar studies of patients (Evarts, 1963, 1964).

When dilantin and other drugs fail to suppress intolerable seizures, a person with really severe epilepsy will consider neurosurgery, during which the source of the seizure is rendered inactive by lesion. In many instances the locus is deep and can be found only by placing electrodes within the brain and then studying the person's brain wave patterns as he sleeps, as he reacts to stress, makes a decision, moves, or perceives clicks, lights, touches. At the Neuropsychiatric Institute of UCLA, where over a dozen such patients have been studied, it has become apparent that nighttime seizures rarely occur during the REM dream phase. Indeed, they occur especially often during stage 2, a period in which the brain waves show a wave form that looks like a wire spindle. The REM state resembles wakefulness in many ways, perhaps imposing the same inhibition upon unruly cells, whose activity erupts in the other stages of sleep—an hypothesis suggested by both the animal study of single cells and the human patient. Until recently, our picture of brain wave patterns from deep sites during specific sleep stages had entirely depended upon implanted animals. We have had no way of knowing whether the hippocampal patterns of cats in REM sleep resembled those of dreaming man. Conversely, we did not know how to interpret unusual brain waves coming from the amygdala of a sleeping epileptic. Were these signs of abnormality or were they also seen in animals during that stage of sleep?

A happy collaboration between the neuropsychiatric hospital and the Space Biology Laboratory of W. Ross Adey has permitted some rapid and invaluable comparisons of humans and primates. One extremely important discovery has centered around activity in the amygdala in man and chimpanzee. A diseased amygdala is often associated with psychomotor epilepsy and is therefore one of the regions that has been probed with electrodes in certain cases. As recent studies have indicated, the sleep of the chimpanzee closely resembles that of man, but some patterns found in the chimp and man have not been seen in other animals, not even monkeys. Thus we must be cautious about generalizing from lower animals to man. One particular observation in the chimpanzee laboratory, however, has clarified a potentially disturbing brain wave pattern seen in epileptic patients. This was a discovery of spindling patterns in the amygdala of a sleeping chimp. When similar bursts emanated from the amygdala of a patient, they might have been mistaken for abnormal signs had the neurosurgeons not known that the same spindling was found in normal chimpanzees. The recent finding, in Dr. Adey's laboratory, that the amygdala may participate in the periodic cycles that form our nightly sleep, points to this frontal region of the brain as a point of particular interest in future studies of sleep, elucidating the mechanisms and the sources of many abnormalities—epilepsy and narcolepsy among them (Adey et al., 1963).

Summary

Sleep disorders and disorders occurring within sleep have provided spore for the scientific hunter, suggesting where to look for the normal mechanisms of sleep, and how they might work. Most disturbed sleep has had its counterpart in a disruption of waking behavior, but only in the last few years have we begun to look at the particular symptoms of troubled sleep for help in diagnosing disturbed behavior and for guidelines in our therapeutic techniques. Insomnia, the most widespread complaint, is a good example. The difference between people who cannot fall asleep, and people who cannot remain asleep may prove to stem from two separate neurophysiological defects—suggesting that the sedatives used for one insomnia may be inappropriate for the other. Hernandez-Peon suggests that emotionally triggered insomnia and inability to fall asleep may spring from an excessive activity within a brain area producing arousal. The inability to sleep through the night, on the other hand, may come from an insufficient chemical supply within a sleep-engendering system in the brain, making it incapable of holding dominance over arousal. Imaginary insomnia, at least insofar as our slim evidence now tells us, may reflect an unusually light sleep or even unusual periodicity among the EEG stages of sleep. When we have learned more about the chemical and neural mechanisms of normal sleep we will be in a better position to treat the many psychological aberrations that accompany these disorders, for sleep disorder does not occur in isolation from the rest of life. Even using today's scanty and recently acquired knowledge of sleep patterns, it has been possible to dispel the fearsome mystery of narcolepsy and outline more sensible procedures for diagnosis and treatment.

Because sleep loss seems to be so generally destructive to the mentally or physically ill, and because of the evidence about the impact of sleep starvation in normal people, it might seem reasonable to prescribe sleep therapy for many disturbances. Sleep therapy has indeed been used in Europe, Russia, and South America for people suffering psychological disturbances, the long periods of sleep induced usually by sedation (Andreev, 1960).

More recently, some investigators have talked of using electrical stimulation instead of sedatives. Sleep has been induced in animals by direct stimulation of certain brain regions, but the evidence from human studies, using surface contacts, has been inconclusive. There has been some confusion about electrosleep, or electronarcosis, and electroanesthesia.

The Russians, using a device similar to an electroanesthesia machine long employed in European animal laboratories, have been credited with producing a sleep with such restful qualities that 2 hours would suffice for 8 hours of sleep. Widely mentioned as a substitute for nightly sleep, the "Elektroson" or similar devices were tried by a few American scientists. The portable device generates low-frequency pulses through electrodes on the eyes and occipital region of the scalp, purportedly to create rhythmic stimulation of the nerve cells in the cerebral cortex. Unfortunately, this situation does not inevitably produce sleep, and although the specifications of the device say that it is intended for inducing sleep electrically, some people in contact with the Russian investigators feel that sleep is a misnomer, and that the device was never intended to induce natural sleep. It is widely used throughout Russia in hundreds of clinics and "sleep stations," for treating headaches, insomnia, certain forms of schizophrenia, epilepsy, stomach ulcers, and neurotic symptoms following head injuries. As a device for "resting the central nervous system," in people with mental illness or psychosomatic disorders, the Russians evidently find this an efficient and successful method. Unfortunately, taking literally the word "sleep" as used in the literature describing the Elektroson, we have concentrated our attention upon the fact that when turned off, the stimulation had not usually left the person in natural sleep. Dr. Sigmund Forster, at New York Downstate Medical Center, found that only half of his subjects fell asleep after electrical stimulation, but patients with muscular disorders experienced relief from symptoms. So few systematic studies have been conducted in this fruitful and interesting area that it has been hard to assess the results. Dr. James A. Lewis at Brooks Air Force Base, San Antonio, Tex., has reviewed much of the electrosleep literature, but this sole review is as yet unpublished.

Electrosleep, as judged by EEGs is not the same as natural sleep, nor, in a more subtle sense, is the prolonged state that is entered under heavy sedation. Recent sleep researches have begun to describe how we alter the natural pattern with various drugs, changing the brain's activity during the several sleep stages and thus, perhaps, affecting many body functions including metabolism. Sleep no longer looks like a unitary process, and sleep disorders appear to arise from many different sources—involving the behavior, training, environment of a person, his body chemistry, and activity at various sites within the brain. Sleep therapy in the future will undoubtedly be tailored to the specific disorder as we discover more about the little-known chemistry of sleep and the way in which body chemicals exert their influence on the brain.

Chapter V.
The Chemistry of Sleep

Whatever elixir of mortal juices helps to prompt a wholesome nightly sleep, it must have been inadequate in 1964, for difficulty in sleeping was a boon to the American drug companies. According to an estimate from one company, private consumers spent about $80 million on sedatives, and this figure included only major prescription sedatives, not over-the-counter drugs, or the sizable purchases of hospitals.

In answer to the public clamor for aid in illness, in transitory or prolonged insomnia, the prescription market offered a sophisticated array by any past standards. Not so long ago the family physician might have prescribed chloral hydrate or "a good stiff drink" in most instances. Today sedation is not so simple (Lester, 1960). The doctor might distinguish between the insomniac who wakens periodically and the person who cannot sleep out the night. One case might warrant a drug that induces rapid sleep onset, and the other a drug that tends to maintain sleep.

Still, the refinement suggested by our present array of drugs does not belie the fact that we continue to remedy sleep disorders in a relatively primitive fashion, and that even what we call insomnia has many roots, whether it be a transient emotional upset, a facet of depression, of old age, or the prelude to acute schizophrenic breakdown. Primarily, these have different metabolic and neural origins, and each demands drugs with particular properties. The brief description of some major sleep disorders in a preceding section may indicate the variety of different things that can go wrong, each hinting at a specific therapy.

In our present and rapidly growing picture of sleep events, it looks as though some people, narcoleptics among them, would be benefited by drugs that increase a particular phase of sleep—the REM period of dreaming. Enuretics and somnambulists appear to need very different pharmaceutical help, perhaps lightening sleep. Others, among them certain depressives and epileptics, may require chemicals that help to stabilize their sleep phases. Schizophrenic patients may need drugs that enhance REM sleep before the omens of acute episodes.

These are, of course, only guesses at the moment, omitting large and unexplored factors from organs such as the liver, glandular systems producing hormones, the role of learned behaviors, and physiological response to the environment. They may, however, illustrate the new approach rapidly entering the treatment of disorders which have, as one noticeable component, symptoms in sleep.

As we begin to face in greater detail the task of countering nature's mischiefs, there are three lines of current research that offer a heartening prospect. Although this is a crude designation, they might be considered together as investigations of the biochemistry of sleep. Using chemical stimulation directly on the brain to elicit sleep and wakefulness, some investigators are attempting to decipher the chemical codes involved in neural activity and determine their anatomical sites. Others have begun to detect chemicals generated within the body or the brain that influence sleep and allied behaviors; the detection of these chemicals offers some hope that we will learn to synthesize and use them. Finally, in studies that have an immediate and practical outcome, some researchers are ferreting out the specific action of the drugs we commonly use, and indeed the effects of diet. The promises and pitfalls of a good deal of this recent work have been reviewed by Arnold Mandell, with reference to the REM state of sleep (Mandell, 1965).

Little enough is known about some of our most common sedatives. However, impact on behavior has been one very useful gauge by which we can distinguish between drugs. During recent years, both sedatives and tranquilizers have been given to patients to help them sleep. At the level of anecdotal observation, there seems to be quite a difference in result. Some clinicians have commented that many patients who come to the clinic asking for sleeping pills, in retrospect seemed to be suffering from the symptoms of incipient mental illness. Given barbiturates for sleep, some may become depressed and even suicidal (Detre et al.).

There seems to be little evidence on this point

at the moment, although a very large number of Americans take their lives each year by swallowing an overdose of sedatives, some of them inadvertently, it is said, while acting in a sedated confusion. There are over 20,000 suicides a year in the United States. A many-faceted study of suicide under the direction of Dr. Edwin S. Shneidman at the Suicide Prevention Center in Los Angeles has already suggested that disturbed sleep may be one of the patterns preceding a suicide attempt, although any influence of specific hypnotic drugs has not yet been revealed.

Drugs are commonly given to institutionalized schizophrenic patients to help them sleep. Ironically, some of the barbiturates that induce sleep in the patient are not therapeutic and actually appear to make him worse. Such has been the observation of an NIH team at St. Elizabeths Hospital in Washington, D.C. What is the meaning of these reports? Some recent studies are beginning to point to differences between barbiturates and tranquilizers.

A series of behavioral studies by Drs. Conan Kornetsky, A. Mirsky, and their associates at Boston University Medical School have been developed in the hope of determining what regions of the brain may be affected by psychoactive drugs. They began by seeking tests that discriminate between drugs that depress attention and those that depress intellectual or cortical activity. Experimentation and long use suggested that a segment of an early IQ test (the Digit Symbol Substitution Test) was a good measure of intellectual functioning, and it was short and easy to administer.

On the test, the subject is given a code by which he matches symbols with numbers on a grid. While sensitive to intellectual performance, this test would not catch lapses of attention. By contrast, the Continuous Performance Test asks the subject to give unremitting attention to a stream of signals, and to respond to certain ones. Here, the omissions of brain-damaged people, or the sleep-starved, or those taking attention-depressing drugs were detected. By using these two tests it was possible to divide psychoactive drugs into those that affect attention and those that affect cortical activity (Mirsky and Kornetsky, 1964).

Two drugs—one a tranquilizer (chlorpromazine) and the other a barbiturate (secobarbital)—seem very similar on the surface, for both produce calm and drowsiness and may leave a slight hangover. Compared by these two tests, however, they are opposites. The tranquilizer reduces attention without damaging intellectual function; the barbiturate, on the other hand, leaves attention undiminished but reduces intellectual performance. This suggests that while both drugs may induce sleep, they may act upon different parts of the brain and perhaps different chemical brain systems. This laboratory is developing apparatus that will make it possible to give these two tests to animals. Once there are parallel tests for drug responses in animals and humans we may be able to test drugs on animals and predict more accurately how they will affect people.

The recent work at Boston University may suggest one reason why schizophrenic patients have benefitted from tranquilizers more than sedatives.

114

Chlorpromazine given to a normal person will depress attention so that he makes many errors on the attention test, as if he had been deprived of sleep. The schizophrenic on the same dose, shows no loss of attention in comparison with his undrugged performance. Perhaps his problem is one of too much neural alertness.

Chlorpromazine helps a schizophrenic patient sleep without intensifying his psychosis. A number of investigators have anticipated that there would be a visible difference in the EEG sleep patterns produced by tranquilizers and sedatives (Freeman et al., 1965). In one study of hallucinating schizophrenics, a St. Elizabeths' team saw that both drugs diminished the amount of REM time in the sleep of psychotic patients but that the barbiturate, phenobarbital, significantly reduced the amount of eye-movements that occurred in the REM stage. Moreover, when the tranquilizer was discontinued, the patient seemed to compensate by increasing REM time, but no such increase followed the removal of phenobarbital.

Well known studies of dream deprivation have suggested that mood and behavior can be harmed by significant reduction in REM sleep, and that a person will compensate with more REM sleep once the deprivation is over. Thus, tentatively, a number of investigators have looked at REM sleep as one kind of index of the effects of drugs or alcohol, permitting at least the loose prediction that continued loss of REM time will have undesirable waking effects.

Alcohol

Alcohol at bedtime does indeed diminish the duration of REM periods during the first hours of sleep. (Gresham et al., 1963). Some years ago, it was speculated that the alcoholic's DT's might be the hallucinations of waking dreams, breaking through after years of continued dream suppression (Greenberg and Pearlman, 1964). A similar conjecture was made about barbiturate psychosis, and more recently about amphetamine psychosis (Kaufman et al., 1964).

Dexedrine

Dexedrine, like alcohol or barbiturates, diminishes the amount of REM sleep. Dexedrine caused restless sleep in volunteers. It could be counteracted by combination with phenobarbital, but the amphetamine continued to suppress dreaming time. When the same subjects were observed on subsequent nights, without medication, they seemed to compensate for the loss, spending more time dreaming than they had before on baseline nights without drugs (Rechtschaffen and Maron, 1964). It was as if they had developed a "need" for REM sleep and this REM hunger, so to speak, may help to explain the psychoses of habitual alcoholics, barbiturate addicts and dexedrine takers. Temporary psychoses are not uncommon after taking these drugs and sometimes the individual may be suffering the effects of all three by the time he comes to a clinic or mental institution.

Dexedrine is currently used for appetite control in daily doses, and the attempt to lose weight in this way can be the start of a vicious circle. While depressing appetite, amphetamines also enhance wakefulness. The weight loser may, therefore,

116

begin taking barbiturates at night in order to sleep. But some sedatives leave a hangover of sluggishness in the morning and therefore the person may increase his dose of dexedrine, only to find that he subsequently needs heavier sedation in order to sleep. Among the patients recovering from such drug psychoses in mental institutions are physicians, whose self-medication escalated in this manner, starting with an effort to lose weight. Have people—on drugs as different as barbiturates and amphetamines—finally reduced their REM time so that an irrepressible need to dream expresses itself during waking and disrupts their behavior?

The answer probably lies in the presently unfolding area of neurophysiology, where it is becoming clear that deprivation of REM sleep can produce strange effects even in cats. Michel Jouvet and his associates of Lyon, by surgically damaging the pontine reticular formation in cats, have removed from the cats' EEG repertoire the pattern corresponding to the REM phase. These cats sleep the sleep of synchronous EEGs but, unless the damage heals and they begin to show the equivalent of REM sleep, they begin to act as if they are hallucinating, and eventually they die (Jouvet, 1960, 1963). Prolonged reduction of REM sleep may indeed play a role in the depressions that often follow in the wake of amphetamines and in the psychotic symptoms of sustained used. The psychological loss of dream content may be some part of the disturbance, and possibly the suppression of a normally recurrent

EEG phase signifies, as well, the suppression of a normal electrochemical sequence, a cycle that may participate in brain and body metabolisms. The evidence, in any event, suggests caution in the use of amphetamines and especially in self-medication.

Barbiturates

A similar caution should apply to the use of barbiturates. Not only have they been shown to reduce REM sleep, and in moderate amounts invoke some intellectual impairment on a behavioral test, but there is some additional data that suggests their mode of action in the brain. Drs. Burton S. Rosner, Truett Allison, and William Goff, used barbiturate anesthesia to filter out (totally obliterate) one portion of the EEG response that the brain will emit after a sensory signal. In some studies subjects were administered an extremely mild electric shock on the skin—during waking, through all stages of sleep, and under drugs. The individual's EEGs, just after the repeated stimulus, were averaged so they could be seen clearly and then analyzed. Although the brain's response, as seen on the EEG, lasted only a few tenths of a second, it combined a sequence of responses from different parts of the brain.

First, roughly speaking, came the response of the specific nerve pathways that conveyed the shock from the wrist to the brain. Then, later in the script, came the emanations from more central regions—diffuse projection systems connected with the cortex. This progression has been ascertained by data too voluminous for enumeration here, but it meant the first letter, so to speak, in the EEG script registered the fact that sensory signals were received in the brain. The subsequent letters signified the activity needed in processing the sensory signal into something meaningful — perception. Under even light barbiturate anesthesia, the response of the specific sensory pathways was if anything enhanced, but the integrative segment of the response was eradicated. This might explain why the EEG would register a pronounced response to a touch, yet the person would feel nothing, and why in surgery there is no awareness of pain, although the brain receives the signals from the body. Even in deepest oblivion of stage 4 sleep the integrative portion of the brain's response registers on the EEG—albeit later and larger than in other stages of sleep.

This suggests that some kind of mentation is occurring during the deepest natural sleep, which may not occur under barbiturates. Current studies may point to the anatomical loci that are inactivated by barbiturate anesthesia and are thought to lie in the diffuse projection systems. Thus, the vanished portions of the EEG response may help to explain several peculiar phenomena that have been noticed in people under barbiturates.

People have shown impaired intellectual capacity on tests. Habitual users of barbiturates, moreover, have reported they sometimes lose their time sense after taking sedation, and will awaken, not knowing the time nor how many pills they have already taken, but will automatically reach for more pills. It seems likely that some of these people have been involuntary suicides. Within the banished portion of the EEG response there may also lie a clue to some of the reported aftereffects of sedation—the so-called hangover. It is still pure conjecture, but not unreasonable to assume that brain activity in sleep plays a role in regulating body functions, metabolic cycles and the progression of biochemical transformations that occur unceasingly throughout life. If barbiturates alter this brain activity, they may be altering at the same time many other physiological functions. The several studies cited here should, if nothing else, indicate that barbiturates do not merely induce sleep—for it now looks as if barbiturate sleep may be missing a component that usually occurs in natural sleep.

Barbiturates are only one class of drugs used in treating sleep disorders. In final analysis a wise use of these—and all centrally active drugs—will depend upon discovering how and where they perform their action within the central nervous system. It will be quite some time before there is such an assay of commonly used drugs, although many investigators have begun using EEG techniques to examine their effects. To a great extent evoked potential studies must be performed upon animals, for only implanted electrodes can reveal changes within small, specific areas deep inside the brain. Walter Rosenblith and his associates, for instance, have used hair-fine electrodes to determine how chloralose and nembutal affect the motor cortex in cats. They would stimulate the paw of the animal and record the EEG response. The brain response would be considerably enhanced by chloralose, but diminished under nembutal. A growing literature of such studies, beyond the scope of this report, is beginning to increase the armamentarium of the pharmacologists, and hopefully will soon allow clinicians to make more fully informed choices in selecting sedation and anesthesia for particular patients. While basic neurophysiological and behavioral studies are beginning to say more about the specific action of drugs, these studies are often inspired by information drawn from clinical studies.

Antidepressants

The treatment of enuresis—bedwetting—has recently evoked some interest in the properties of imipramine, an antidepressant. Drs. Keith S. Ditman and Alvin F. Poussiant, at the UCLA Neuropsychiatric Institute, have administered this drug to children who were incorrigible bedwetters and found that 85 percent of their volunteers stopped bedwetting. On the other hand, they also became somewhat irascible. This is an interesting finding. The investigators believed that imipramine enabled some bladder relaxation, and therefore greater fluid capacity, but also that it lightened sleep, acting as a mild stimulant, so that the child was able to awaken when he needed to go to the bathroom.

Two or three years earlier Dr. Roy Whitman and his associates at the University of Cincinnati had shown that imipramine very significantly reduced REM sleep time in adults. In a study of dream content, under several drugs, the one very consistent finding was that people taking imipramine reported a striking number of hostile dreams (Whitman et al., 1961). The irritability of the children taking the drug might conceivably be related to the reduction of REM sleep. But this does not explain hostile dream content, or the fact that the drug has an enlivening effect on depressed patients. The observations suggest that the EEG phases of sleep may be regulated by neural centers also involved in invoking moods, and that the processes affecting sleep affect emotional tone as well. If mood and sleep are interlocked in the same processes, a certain degree of activation might generate cheer, although a greater degree of excitation might become manifest as irritability. The impact of a drug undoubtedly depends upon the initial state of the person—and a depressed person may indeed require artificial excitation in order to rise to a normal level, whereas a normal adult or child might be subjected to overexcitement by the same dose.

Questions about brain-metabolism have been raised by the effects of another antidepressant, "Iproniazid." In 1957, Dr. Nathan Kline of Rockland State Hospital began testing ambulatory depressed patients with this drug. After a time the report was made, several such patients had such reduced desire to sleep that they had been averaging three to four hours a night for well over a year (Kline, 1961). Iproniazid, and other monoamine oxidase inhibitors tested since, may enhance the action of serotonin and the stimulant norepinephrine in the brain, possibly promoting more efficient brain metabolism (Murray, in press; Bailey, et al., 1959).

The EEG pattern of normal sleep—as roughly judged from the hundreds of nights on record—

has become one of the rulers against which drug effects are measured, and particular emphasis has been placed upon the amount of REM sleep. Many drugs suppress REM dreaming. At the same time current studies of narcoleptics, of drug psychotics, and alcoholics suggest that these people need a drug that increases dreaming. Before therapists can prescribe more dreaming, such a pharmaceutical must be found.

LSD-25

The hallucinogenic properties of LSD-25 have suggested that it might increase nightly dreamtime. In an initial study, using cats as subjects, Dr. J. A. Hobson of NIH found no increase of REM time. Instead, the LSD had an arousing effect, so much so that it deterred the animals from sleeping (Hobson, 1964). This was a discouraging result, but it underlined a difficulty that must be particularly common in research on psychoactive drugs. As more recent studies have pointed out, dosage is a critical factor. In small enough doses, LSD appears to have the dream enhancing property that was expected.

A team working at the Columbia University School of Medicine has succeeded in greatly increasing the length of particular REM periods at the height of the drug's action (Muzio, Roffwarg, and Kaufman, 1964). This was a human study, and the 12 volunteers were studied over a year. At first the attempts seemed doubtful. The dose had to be modified for each individual. This adjustment sometimes took 10 successive attempts, and each session had to be spaced long enough after the previous trial so that all traces of the

123

drug would have worn off.

The dosages were very small, ranging between 0.16–0.73 mcg. per kilogram of body weight, about the equivalent of one five-hundredth of an aspirin. A few volunteers showed a spectacular increase in total REM sleep. One subject, given his tiny amount of LSD, tripled the length of his second REM period. Several others doubled their first or second REM periods. It has been postulated that dreaming may be triggered by a neurochemical that acts upon the brain stem reticular and pontine-limbic systems. Perhaps LSD acts upon these centers and bears some family resemblance to an intrinsic dream triggering chemical. Since LSD has increased REM sleep in humans, we can now hope to develop a drug therapy for people who need to "dream more," perhaps one that can be used in conjunction with the numerous hypnotics that we now know suppress REM sleep.

During the last year another subject in another laboratory responded to LSD with an increase in REM sleep (Green, in press). The investigator observed that the person also showed somewhat more body movement than usual and more vocalization in sleep. The dosage in this instance (300 mcg.) was truly huge by comparison with that of the previous study. Underlying the problem of dose adjustment to an individual are a host of complicated factors, his constitution, his personality, his metabolism, and many others. The great variation in the human population makes it difficult to generalize at an early stage of exploration and predict how any specific individual will react to a given amount of the chemical. Similar variation has been observed in laboratory animals and has recently become the focus of study (Brown and Shryne, 1964).

Some of the changes in brain function caused by LSD and other hallucinogens have been examined in EEG studies of animals and humans (Adey et al., 1962; Chapman et al., 1962). These are among the studies offering clues to the regions of the higher mammal brain that generate hallucination and may help us determine how the brain performs as we hallucinate or dream. Surely, investigations of "dream enhancing chemicals" are bound to increase because of their potential medical benefits and because of the light they may shed upon the nature of the REM cycle itself.

LSD is a known hallucinogen, but another chemical that can act as a depressant, reserpine, has also increased REM time in people although it has had an opposite effect upon cats (Hartmann, 1965). Reserpine releases a natural neurochemical, serotonin, whose possible role in sleep and dreaming is currently causing some interest.

A Possible Hypnotoxin

In the pursuit of chemicals with special and remarkable properties—like dream enhancement—there has been a growing interest in some compounds that are produced within the body. By what chemicals does the body produce sleep? Where are they manufactured and stored? How do they metabolize? We might achieve a truly refined control of sleep disorders if we could simulate the body's own biochemical behavior. Toward this ultimate goal, a number of current researches have been exploring the properties of sex hormones, of gamma-hydroxybutyrate, a metabolite of GABA, and the cerebrospinal fluid of animals in various states of sleep, sleep starvation, or dream starvation.

In the early part of our century it was widely conjectured that sleep resulted from a toxin, perhaps generated by the fatigued body. In 1910, a "hypnotoxin" was reported by Legendre and Pieron (Kleitman, 1963). Cerebrospinal fluid from a sleep-deprived dog caused drowsiness and other symptoms of sleeplessness in a normally rested animal while spinal fluid from a rested animal had no such effect. Quite a number of related experiments followed, but there was a seemingly insuperable difficulty: animals gave a depressed reaction to injection, whatever the injection contained. The idea that sleep could be transmitted from a sleeping animal to an alert one by some body chemical manufactured during sleep was in general disrepute for some time.

Recently, however, the trick seems to have been accomplished by Drs. M. Monnier and L. Hosli of the University of Basel, Switzerland. A dialysate of brain blood from a sleeping rabbit caused sleep in an alert one (Monnier, 1964). Moreover, a dialysate of the venous cerebral blood from an alert creature produced arousal in a sleeping recipient. Since the donor animals were put to sleep by electrical stimulation to the thalamus and alerted by stimulation of the reticular formation, sham stimulations were used as controls. Dialysate of sham stimulation produced quite different results in the receiving animals. This is perhaps a first step in discovering a general hypnotic within the cerebral blood of a sleeping creature. Dialysis, a process of filtering liquid through a membrane, removed the heavy colloidal particles from the blood—but the remaining mixture is complicated, indeed, and we are a long way from knowing which compounds may be the active ones. Still the search has a great appeal, for the isolating of a natural and general hypnotic could help us to unravel the chemical process of sleep and offer sensitive control over sleep.

In a related vein, Dr. W. C. Dement and his associates at Stanford University have been attempting to find a postulated neurochemical that may trigger the dreaming phase of sleep. A description of this work will make more sense within the context of a section on REM sleep.

Although searching the cerebrospinal fluid or brain tissue for signs of a particular chemical effect may seem horrendously difficult—worse than looking for a needle in a haystack—there is a certain advantage to finding an effect within spinal fluid, an advantage that does not obtain if the chemical is found elsewhere in the body. If substances that engender dreaming or sleep can be detected within spinal fluid, these will be distinct from other body chemicals with the same effect. One reason is the well-known blood-brain barrier that prevents many substances in the blood from entering the brain. The existence of this barrier is well documented, but its nature remains something of a mystery. Sometimes it appears to be a matter of delay, preventing a rapid exchange from the blood to the brain. Even when a compound produces its effect—sleep, or dreaming—after direct injection into the brain, there remains some question about the form in which it naturally works in the body. Chemicals in the body can undergo a chain of transformations with lightning speed: Does the injected form of a chemical act directly upon the brain cells, or is the effective chemical some metabolite? This prelude may outline the background of a controversy that surrounds one of the exciting new compounds in the realm of sleep.

Gamma-hydroxybutyrate

Gamma-hydroxybutyrate may be called the center of the interest, one of a family of structurally related compounds that have been shown to produce REM sleep, or paradoxical sleep as it is known in animals. It has been used as an anesthetic and has no hangover effect, and is being investigated as a possible "hibernation" drug for man in space. It is related to a naturally occurring body chemical (Gamma-amino-butyric-acid) GABA, and controversy rages about the question: Does this chemical, or its lactone form, exist in the brain or body organs in enough quantity to become a natural hypnotic? The answer may be that it metabolizes so rapidly that it is generated only on demand. Drs. Samuel Bessman and Sandra Skolnik at the University of Maryland have found that injection of the lactone form is particularly sleep-inducing and that lactone may be produced from a known body chemical by a special enzyme in the liver—perhaps a clue to the drowsiness, depression, and even coma that sometimes attend liver disease (Bessman and Skolnik,

1964). Other investigators at Yale University have not been able to find it in the blood or brains of laboratory animals by gas chromatography, possibly because its metabolism is too rapid (Giarman and Roth, 1964). GHB, injected into animals, can be detected in their breath seconds later.

While the controversy over its endogenous origins goes undecided, Gamma-hydroxybutyrate will continue to be the focus of excited study. At the University of Maryland, Drs. Robert Vidaue, Gerald Klee, and Russell Monroe are investigating its effect, in different doses, on people. So far they have found that it produces an EEG pattern similar to that of chloralose—with a quick appearance of paroxysmal theta and delta waves preceding sleep. Given intravenously, another form of this chemical—sodium 4-hydroxy-butyrate—produces sleep within 10 minutes. In France, the compound has been used as an anesthetic in many thousands of people, but in combination with morphine or other analgesic.

An anesthetic with no hangover can be a mixed blessing. When the drug has worn off the animal or person will quickly awaken, and move around. He will not show the sluggishness caused by barbiturates. On the other hand, the groggy aftermath of the barbiturate may dull the experience of pain. After GHB anesthesia, the pain occurs as rapidly as awakening, a reason for administering an analgesic.

EEG studies with animals have indicated why these two kinds of anesthesia produce such different effects. The clue can be seen in the brainwave response to a stimulus. During barbiturate anesthesia the cortical or integrative part of the EEG response is obliterated, although the response representing reception of sensory signals actually appears enhanced. Under barbiturates, it would seem, the sensory signals get into the brain but are never transformed into perception. Under GHB or related compounds the opposite seems to occur. The sensory signals do not seem to enter the brain and the integrative functions remain undiminished. Thus, the one appears to depress functions necessary to awareness, the other to censor the actual input of the senses.

Herein lies the key to some of the excitement about this new family of chemicals. Unlike the barbiturate, it leaves integrative-cortical functions intact. Judging from EEG responses, it would seem to produce an effect in the brain that is congruent with the response pattern of REM sleep. The EEG responses give the signs that it inhibits sensory input, without diminishing integrative functions. This is exactly the kind of EEG response pattern observed many times by many investigators in subjects during REM (paradoxical) sleep. The property of censoring incoming sense signals while leaving integrative functions alone may be an important attribute in any hypnotic that will not suppress dreaming.

Experiments with gammabutyrolactone have shown that it will induce paradoxical sleep in cats. This finding about this chemical and some of its related compounds has prompted considerable study. In point of fact, the studies began several years ago in Lyon, in both acute and chronic cats. In an acute experiment the procedure necessarily terminates the life of the animal, whereas the so-called chronic animal may be observed in the laboratory for weeks, months, or years following the experimental procedure (Jouvet et al., 1961). More recently acute experiments of the same sort have been performed in Tokyo (Matsuzaki et al., 1964). Intravenous injections of sodium butyrate and related compounds were used to induce paradoxical sleep in cats whose brains had been transected at the mesencephalon as well as in intact animals. The chemicals elicited paradoxical sleep in cats with midbrain transections, as well as in intact animals.

Whatever its usefulness as a tool in deciphering the mechanism of REM dreaming, this new family of compounds holds great promise as a hypnotic that does not depress REM sleep. Indeed, its extraterrestrial value may cause more study than its potential usefulness here on earth. It appears to be one candidate for producing hibernation during long space flights. If there is to be such a thing as drug-induced hibernation for space travel or medical purposes, surely today's evidence indicates that the drug should not cause REM loss. Space scientists have been investigating 4-hydroxybutyrate. The compound elicits a significant drop in body temperature—about 3°—which is greater than the normal nightly decline. At the same time, oxygen consumption is decreased. Studies of humans in prolonged 4-HB sleep may tell whether the overall effect is that of natural sleep.

The ideal of course would be a drug that permitted us to produce sleep in the same way the body does. There are many reasons for suspecting that the body triggers sleep biochemically, and the search for these chemicals is not at all new. There have been attempts to find a hypnotic chemical produced by muscular activity, by wastes, many attempts based upon the logic that one should find a "fatigue" substance generated by waking activity. These attempts have not yet succeeded, and today experimenters have begun to think that they may not be searching for just one substance. There might be several chemical mechanisms stemming from different metabolic chains, having different effects even though the net results might look like the same behavior—sleep. Recent experiments begin to suggest that indeed slow-wave sleep and REM sleep may be influenced, and perhaps triggered, by totally different chemicals.

The suspicion that two different chemicals may trigger sleep and REM sleep has been phrased informally for several years, and it is heightened by evidence from the diverse researches of Dr. Michel Jouvet, of Lyon, France, and Dr. Werner Koella, of the Worcester Foundation for Experimental Biology, in Shrewsbury, Mass.

Reserpine

The French researchers have looked closely at the sleep of cats following an injection of reserpine. This compound is a derivative of Rauwolfia or snakeroot, an ancient Indian remedy that has been used extensively in modern form to calm people in states of intense emotional disorder and to lower blood pressure in hypertensives. Reserpine reduces slow wave sleep, and its impact upon

132

the paradoxical phase of sleep in cats might be said to resemble a sledgehammer. After a single injection of reserpine, paradoxical sleep would decline, disappearing altogether for 5 days. This remarkable effect strongly suggested that reserpine must inactivate brain centers or brain chemicals that are essential to paradoxical sleep.

Reserpine is known to reduce the content of serotonin in the brain and to affect other brain chemicals. A number of these chemicals were subsequently administered to determine whether they counteracted the impact of reserpine on paradoxical sleep. A cat was given reserpine, and then an injection of 5-hydroxytryptophane (5–HTP). This is a substance known to precede serotonin in the metabolic cycle. Serotonin is 5–hydroxytryptamine, and 5–HTP is a substance from which it is built. An injection of 5–HTP should have restored serotonin in the reserpine-injected cat. If an increase in serotonin were crucial to paradoxical sleep, then it should have reappeared. Not so. The cat now showed a normal pattern of slow wave sleep but not a sign of the paradoxical REM phase. However, if the shot of reserpine were followed by an injection of dopa, REM sleep did reappear.

Dopa

Dopa is a precursor of noradrenalin, a substance produced in neural tissue throughout the body and brain. When dopa was administered to a cat that never received reserpine its effect was striking. Given to a normal cat, dopa increased the animal's paradoxical sleep. However, if a normal and unmedicated cat were given 5–HTP instead, its paradoxical REM sleep was depressed. This series of findings suggested that paradoxical sleep might be dependent upon chemicals related to adrenalin and noradrenalin, but not to serotonin.

Serotonin

Serotonin would appear to play a role in producing slow wave sleep. As usual, in science, a long history of researches into the effects of serotonin on blood pressure and many brain functions preceded the studies that implicate serotonin in slow wave sleep (Koella, et al., 1960, 1961, 1963, 1965; Koella, 1962). In recent researches the investigators noticed that serotonin was producing some peculiar effects on brainwaves (Koella et al., 1965). When injected into the carotid artery of an immobilized or anesthetized cat, serotonin promptly produced an arousal reaction. This brief EEG arousal pattern was then followed by 15–20 minutes of slow waves and sleep spindles, and the large spindling EEG pattern known as a recruiting response.

The recruiting response has drawn interest because it may be related to the normal EEG spindles seen in sleep. Experimenters have found that they could obtain this EEG recruiting response by electrically stimulating the medial aspects of the thalamus. Sleep has also been produced by stimulating this same thalamic region (Akert, et al., 1952). Perhaps it is not surprising that an injection of a chemical might produce both the EEG recruiting response and brainwaves typical of sleep. The experimenters found it curious, however, that the same chemical first produced an arousal response, and wondered if they were seeing reactions from two distinct portions of the brain.

This hunch was borne out by the experiments that followed. The brain stem of a cat was surgically transected so that the effect of serotonin was only apparent on the anterior portion: now the animal showed the brain waves of arousal but there was no sleep. This implied that serotonin was inducing sleep by affecting the posterior brain stem, at the very base of the brain. The experimenters began exploring a very small structure at the base of the brain stem, the area postrema, which might be described as a gateway region to the central nervous system. When this small area was destroyed in cerebellectomized cats, the serotonin injection continued to cause arousal and not sleep. The researchers now zeroed in on the area postrema.

This region has been known to accept serotonin and other similar chemicals, i.e., it has no blood-brain barrier. It now seemed to be the specific neural receptor site on which serotonin acted to facilitate sleep. Instead of surgically destroying the area postrema the experimenters took their next step to nullify the action of serotonin here by chemically blocking the receptor site and thus preventing the sleep response. LSD and other chemicals block the action of serotonin, which is a neural transmitter. When one of these blocking agents was applied to the area postrema an injection of serotonin caused the EEGs of arousal, but not sleep. On the other hand, whenever serotonin was placed in the area postrema of an intact cat the EEG's gave only the signs of sleep, not arousal.

Serotonin seemed a likely candidate as a body-generated chemical that induces sleep. Surely if a body chemical were responsible for inducing sleep one might expect it to act at the base of the brain near the spinal cord. There is one interesting fact, however. Serotonin does not pass through the blood-brain barrier. Thus it could not directly reach with its effects deep into the brain stem. An exploration of the area postrema, where serotonin is received, may however explain how serotonin could cause a hypnogenic response in the rest of the brain. The area postrema is connected by dendrites to an adjacent area within the brain, the nucleus of the tractus solitarius which is probably not directly permeable to serotonin, but may receive its effects through the dendrites linking it with the area postrema.

The action of serotonin as described here may illustrate what is often referred to as the triggering action—or triggering chemical. Serotonin may act as a neutral trigger. It stimulates receptors within the area postrema, which, in turn, stimulates cells in an adjacent nucleus tractus solitarius, perhaps causing a neutral chain reaction whose consequence we know as sleep (Koella, et al., 1965).

The indication that serotonin can induce sleep by its action upon a brainstem structure does not eliminate the possibility that other body chemicals also participate in producing natural sleep. Serotonin is chemically like a hormone, and acts as a neutral transmitter over very short distances. Other investigators have been looking at the effects of sex

136

hormones for an elucidation of the natural sleep process.

Hormones

Unnatural sleepiness, or at any rate excessive sleepiness, is the accompaniment of numerous disorders, but also occurs in normal people who are undergoing changes in body chemistry. In a book called "Pregnancy and Birth," A. F. Guttmacher has described one of the most common of sleep disorders. "In some women, one of the earliest signs of pregnancy is an overpowering sleepiness. Sleeping late in the morning and napping in the afternoon do not prevent the pregnant young wife from yawning in her husband's face and from dozing even at her own dinner parties. This excessive need for sleep disappears after the first few months." Although the soporific serenity of a pregnant woman bears no resemblance to the blankness of an epileptic seizure, or the catalepsy of a narcoleptic, the catatonic state of a schizophrenic, or the anesthesia state, there may be a chemical link between them. Somnolence, anesthesia, and convulsions may all be produced by different concentrations of progesterone, the hormone secreted in large quantities by pregnant woman. Progesterone, indeed, is only one of the hormones known to produce an anesthetic state, and some have been used as an anesthetic.

Drs. George M. Ling and Gunnar Heuser are currently collaborating at UCLA on a study of the effects of several steroid hormones on the central nervous system. They have shown that two precursors of hormones (dehydroepiandrosterone, and II-desoxycortisol) will produce sedation in low dosages, while high doses invoke seizures and convulsions. By administering finely graded doses they hope to determine whether steroids will produce sleep in the amounts secreted by the body. A connection between sex hormones and sleepiness should not seem surprising, for it is observed frequently without any reflection, in the aftermath of lovemaking, people tend to fall asleep.

Hormones appear not only to elicit sleep, but perhaps also to change its quality by influencing the EEG phases and duration. Drs. Ling and Heuser have observed that cats sleep a good deal longer given progesterone, than if they are sedated with compounds that resemble the neurochemicals serotonin and acetylcholine. Moreover, the sleep induced with progesterone is distinguished by ample episodes of paradoxical sleep. In studies of eight pregnant cats they found that the incidence of paradoxical sleep increased as pregnancy progressed toward delivery, and during the brief post partum interval after delivery the cats also showed frequent periods of paradoxical sleep. There may indeed be some truth to the old wives' tale that a woman dreams a lot when pregnant. The story does not seem to be a simple one, however, and an increase of progesterone should not be expected to produce an orgy of dreams. Under some circumstances it may do the opposite.

Enovid, a combination of a progestergen derivative and an estrogen, both female sex hormones, prevents ovulation. One sign of its antifertility effect has been that it delays or suppresses signs of dreaming normally seen in a female rabbit just following coitus. Ordinarily the fertile rabbit will quickly lapse into sleep, soon showing EEG signs of paradoxical sleep, but if her production of ovulatory hormones has been blocked, the familiar EEG patterns of paradoxical sleep will not occur. This index of fertility—and method of quickly detecting an antifertility compound—was discovered by Dr. Charles Sawyer and his associates at UCLA as they explored the relation between the sex steroids, brain activity, and fertility. Here, paradoxical sleep played the role of a key into the brain processes that govern sexual behavior and reproductive capacity (Kanematsu and Sawyer, 1963; Kawakami and Sawyer, 1959, 1962; Sawyer, 1961, 1963).

The solution to the world's crushing problems of overpopulation may hinge upon some of these recent discoveries about the neurochemistry of fertility, among them the finding that Enovid and other steroids that block ovulation act upon the central nervous system. The impact of steroids on ovulation had to be reinterpreted in the early 1960's when Drs. Sawyer and Kawakami knit together their diverse findings on many species, showing, among other things, that these compounds depressed the likelihood of paradoxical sleep following sexual stimulation. Rabbits were used a great deal because they are reflex ovulators; that is, ovulation is induced by coitus, whether real, artificial, or performed by brain stimulation. The characteristic afterreaction to coitus is unambiguous, even without EEGs, for in slow-wave sleep the rabitt's ears remain erect, but when paradoxical sleep begins they suddenly lose muscle tone and droop. This reaction was probed by the injection of pituitary hormones and by direct stimulation of the hypothalamus, which could produce the rabbit's afterreaction. In tests of many hormones and other compounds, it became clear that barbiturates, the tranquilizer chlorpromazine, and morphine had a pronounced effect upon the afterreaction of the rabbit—suggesting that they may block the nervous activation of the pituitary gland in releasing ovulatory hormones. In this regard, it is interesting to note that morphine addicts tend to be infertile, and female addicts generally have irregular menstrual cycles.

In a long series of studies with various techniques, using steroids directly upon the brain or surgical lesions in the hypothalamus, it became clear that the brain centers controlling sexual behavior and those controlling pituitary hormonal function were quite discrete in the rabbit and sexual behavior could be independent of influences on fertility. Thus, the brain seemed to contain a fertility center, sensitive to steroids, which would induce ovulation after electrical stimulation, but if damaged, would cause gonadal atrophy. The location of this center (the posterior basal tuber of the hypothalamus) in a brain region known to play a large role in emotion, may enable us to determine how emotions—mood, anxiety, and stress, affect fertility. If stress hormones, and neurohumors of emotion act upon this region to block fertility, we may learn how to treat some of the perplexing cases of sterility for which people seek clinical aid. A classic instance of what seems to be "emotional" infertility is that of the couple who cannot conceive, but who do, indeed, begin producing children shortly after adopting a child.

The explorations outlined so scantily here, raise important and as yet unanswered questions about the influence of hormones on mood and sleep. Quite beyond supplying an index by which anti-ovulatory drugs can be screened, the paradoxical sleep of the postcoital rabbit has instigated many assays of sleep patterns and hormones. Dr. Kawakami has shown that an animal going into estrus has an increasing ratio of paradoxical to slow-wave sleep. Female rabbits, given the male hormone, testosterone, will not show paradoxical sleep after mating, nor will the normal male. But a castrated male, given the female hormone estrogen, will show this sleep symptom following electrical stimulation of the septum (Kawakami and Sawyer, 1962). What is the relation between the sex steroids and paradoxical sleep? Do they suppress dreaming in human beings? Could steroids and other antifertility agents act upon the lateral hypothalamus to affect mood and incur subtle personality changes?

Further explorations in this direction may help to explain emotional differences between the sexes. Moreover, they may help to explain psychological phenomena that are clearly linked to sexual periodicities, such as the depressions and exhilarations of women at the onset of menstruation and during the postparturitional days. In pilot studies with cats, Dr. Sawyer believes he has seen changes in temperament after hypothalamic lesions that block ovulation. Patterns of sleep, showing us something of the integration of the nervous system

141

by which we can compare normal and altered states, have provided a new tool for what promises to be an even more important skein to unwind in a world where fertility is likely to be controlled with drugs.

No extensive EEG studies have yet been conducted upon pregnant women, or women taking Enovid. The widespread testing and use of Enovid for birth control, and, in higher doses, for the treatment of a pelvic disease associated with infertility, have enabled clinicians to observe some psychological effects. Many women have discontinued the use of Enovid because it makes them feel depressed or irritable. When heavy therapeutic doses were tried for the purposes of advancing fertility among wives of armed services personnel, temporary psychosis occurred in about 4 percent. Whether these symptoms could be detected or even anticipated by changes in EEG sleep patterns is still an open question.

We have known for almost a decade that sex hormones can act directly upon neural tissue. However, nobody will forget the startling demonstration that a male hormone, placed within a particular brain region, engenders the confusing result of maternal nesting behavior in male rats (Fisher, A. E.). So we have, by implication, the problem that we are not just dealing with neurochemistry as we explore hormonal effects, but also anatomical organization and the responsiveness of specific areas to specific chemicals. Do steroid hormones naturally act upon certain brain regions— or do steroids act as a trigger for other brain chemicals? The EEG patterns of sleep are being used in researches to answer this question.

A great many factors have encouraged the suspicion that the sex hormones play an important role in sleep patterns, in mood, and in dreaming. The fact that adults begin to show a decline of REM sleep after age 40, is in itself suggestive. A recent study of the sleep of five women has added to this evidence. Women undergo cyclic hormonal fluctuations, marked by menstruation, and also by variations in mood that are so severe in a small percentage as to approach mild psychosis and demand medical aid. If hormonal changes were reflected in sleep, one would expect to see cyclic changes in women. In an initial study, changes have been observed, especially in increases of dream time falling toward the middle or end of the monthly cycle (Hartmann, 1965). Curiously enough, these periods of higher dreaming coincide with periods of anxiety and sometimes depression.

Dr. David Hamburg and M. Dallman at Stanford University Medical School have been injecting progesterone directly into the hypothalamus in rabbits, but analyses of brain tissue have not yet revealed whether the hormone acts directly on the brain. Why would hormonal levels affect sleep, and even induce sleep, if they do not act within the brain?

Acetylcholine and Noradrenalin

A number of investigators have speculated that substances such as hormones affect the levels of two important brain amines which do, in turn, produce sleep or arousal. Current research by Drs. Ling, Fisher, Hernandez-Peon, and numerous investigators in other areas of neurochemistry may show us that the brain operates on a chemical code, and that two of its principal code chemicals are acetylcholine and noradrenalin. These are found throughout the nervous system. They are produced at nerve ends in the body and brain, and appear to play an important role in transmitting nerve impulses from one cell to another. They appear, additionally, to play an essential part in the homeostasis of the body, maintaining the equilibrium of the autonomic nervous system, stabilizing heart rate, or stomach motility.

Dr. Ling postulates that these two chemicals play a homeostatic, or a balancing role within the central nervous system as well. Noradrenalin is related to dexedrine, one of the amines of the nervous system that promotes alertness, and acts as a psychic energizer. In excess, this amine may also bring anxiety, restlessness, and the mental states associated with insomnia. On the other hand, as he has demonstrated with cats, acetylcholine produces somnolence in the same brain sites where noradrenalin evokes arousal. Perhaps this acetylcholine, in large concentration, invokes apathy and even depression. These two chemicals may be natural components of sleep and arousal, and small increases in their concentration might transform mere arousal into acute anxiety and turn sleep into depression. Such speculations are emphatically tentative at the moment, but they are bound to provide a rich inspiration for research— for they suggest techniques by which we may discover the close biochemical ties between sleep, hormones, and mental illness.

Right now, anyway, it looks as if there are two major chemical systems at work in causing nervous tissue to perform. The cholinergic system may be inhibitory. In other words, acetylcholine may be the neurochemical that excites brain cells that cause sleep, or the cessation of an activity, but this inhibitory work does not go on infinitely, because another chemical, cholinesterase, acts like a brake halting the potent action of acetylcholine. Cells instigating arousal, or other specific excitation, may be activated by the neural stimulants of the adrenergic system—noradrenalin and adrenalin. Presumably these also have a chemical brake, but little is known about their metabolism at present. This is a vastly oversimplified view, yet it may provide a kind of primitive map to some of the basic research currently probing relationships between sleep and mental illness and their biochemical nature.

Some investigators have been systematically probing a particular region of the brain. Dr. Nathaniel Buchwald and his associates at UCLA, for instance, have been stimulating one brain center and charting the associated behavioral changes and EEG patterns at other sites in the brain (Heuser et al., 1961). This is an anatomically distinct island, located under the cortex, in the forepart of the brain—the caudate nucleus. Here is the largest supply of cholinesterase stored in the brain, a braking chemical for acetylcholine and the nervous activity it incites. When cholinesterase is destroyed in this area and electric stimulation is gently applied, the animal suffers tremors or epileptiform seizures. Because the caudate nucleus is one of the brain's largest storehouses of important chemicals, among them dopa and dopamine, it may offer some clues about the neurochemistry of parkinsonian tremors, epileptic fits, and schizophrenia.

Chemical Brain Mapping

Following another approach, some scientists have been using acetylcholine and noradrenalin directly upon the brain, in a manner analogous to electrical stimulation, thus learning which brain systems respond to cholinergic chemicals and which respond to adrenergic stimulation. The implement, chemical stimulation, has had an extremely important impact upon our understanding of the anatomy of sleep.

Using brain chemicals as his probe, Dr. Raul Hernandez-Peon, and his colleagues, working largely in Mexico City, have shown that sleep is promoted and regulated by a large system of brain cells, sweeping from the frontal regions down to the brain stem with centers in the thalamus and cerebellum. During the last decade there was a growing confusion about the brain centers that, upon stimulation, caused an animal to sleep. There were so many of them—electrical stimulation in the frontal regions, or caudal regions, in the thalamus and hypothalamus—and all seemed to invoke the well-known EEG patterns and behavior of sleep. This electrical brain mapping had begun with the pioneering work of W. R. Hess of Zurich, who had produced eating, rage, and other behavior by delivering mild electrical pulses to the brains of animals. Electrical stimulation of the brain became a valuable tool and was widely used.

In their memorable experiments of the late 1940's and early 1950's, Moruzi and Magoun excited the world of brain research with their discovery that stimulation to the reticular formation led to arousal and wakefulness. Here was evidence of an arousal center in the brain. Logically enough, sleep was considered to be the mere lack of reticular activity—a passive state, brought about by default so to speak. Today, however, sleep does not look like the consequence of a lack of activity in the brain, but the result of activity within a specific neural system, a system that actively inhibits arousal. This was the assumption on which Dr. Hernandez-Peon and his associates set to work, at a time, it should be added, when the outcome was quite uncertain. They sought to locate a topographical map, if possible, showing where and perhaps how the brain produces what we know as sleep.

Although they set out, using brain stimulation as their main experimental probe, on an expedition to map the uncharted sleep system, and were not primarily interested in its biochemical properties, they came to rely heavily upon chemical stimulation. One reason was the diffuseness of electrical stimulation. If a pulse were delivered to neural cells within a particular system, it might cause activity among cells adjacent but outside of that system. Any neuron might be activated, inadvertently. For refined brain mapping, then, psychologists and neurophysiologists wanted a more selective method, a stimulus that would spark only the cells involved in a particular activity. They tried using the chemicals known to modify synaptic transmissions in nerves throughout the body, among them, acetylcholine and noradrenalin.

Animals were implanted with fine electrodes for EEG recording and sometimes for stimulation or the creation of small lesions. Similarly they were implanted with fine cannulae, hollow guide-shafts through which a tiny chemical crystal could be tamped to the nerve cells. Like electrodes, these cannulae could be left in place comfortably, and the experimental animals had freedom of movement and a relatively normal laboratory existence. A fine screw threading would permit the experimenter to stimulate a locus, and move the cannula a millimeter at a time through seven depths of tissue.

Cats were the primary experimental animal in mapping the sleep system, and acetylcholine has been the chemical that stimulates hypnogenic centers in this animal, putting it to sleep. Species differ, however; if you stimulate a rat brain, in roughly the same pathway that elicits sleep in cats, acetylcholine will evoke thirst and drinking. However, apply noradrenalin to certain parts of the rat brain, corresponding to the regions in which acetylcholine produces sleep in cats—and noradrenalin evokes sleep in the rat (Fisher, 1964).

The hypnogenic response of the cat to acetylcholine was supported by a few simple experiments. If the animal were given atropine, or another chemical that blocks acetylcholine, then electrical stimulation failed to produce sleep in the very spot where it had formerly evoked sleep. An animal, put to sleep by several brief electrical

148

stimulations to a brain locus, then injected with atropine, remained wakeful through repeated electrical stimulation. Presumably, the missing element was the blocked, biochemical action of acetylcholine (Hernandez-Peon, 1963).

Nerve impulses can be stimulated by electric shock and detected by electric sensing devices, but the nerve impulse itself is not like an electric current passing along a wire. Rather, it results from a biochemical change in the membrane surrounding a nerve cell, a movement of ions, electrically charged particles that follow the release of a chemical transmitter from a neighboring neuron. Electrical stimulation, therefore, causes biochemical action. It is not like feeding current into an electronic machine. The electrical stimulation that was producing sleep must have caused a release of acetylcholine at the synapses of the sleep neurons, a release that was blocked by atropine, with the consequence that acetylcholine no longer acted as a biochemical transmitter and the sleep neurons were no longer activated.

Using acetylcholine and electrical probes, in countless experiments on hundreds of cats, it was found that there was indeed a hypnogenic pathway, beginning far forward in the frontal and temporal lobes, with a center in the thalamus, and extending downward toward the spinal cord. Lesion experiments demonstrated that this cholinergic pathway has both an ascending and descending route. Messages are borne downward from the cortex and frontal brain regions to the brain stem, and also upwards from the spinal cord—inhibiting the vigilance system of the brain stem.

149

(Hernandez-Peon, 1963).

Most people have noticed that all sleep is not alike—it occurs faster on some occasions, like the sudden dropping of a shade. It differs in quality. Some of the experiments suggest why this may be. The same crystals of acetylcholine, touched to different brain sites, produced somewhat different results. Ordinarily, if a cat is placed in a laboratory cage and left alone, it will settle down and fall asleep in 15–30 minutes. When acetylcholine was injected into the preoptic region of the hypothalamus, a waking cat fell asleep in 2–5 minutes. The same stimulation to another hypnogenic area, however, caused sleep in 22 seconds.

Films of this study convey the instantaneousness of the effect. A cat, in the midst of eating, received stimulation in the sleep-circuit, and literally fell asleep so fast that his head dropped into his food dish. Speed of sleep onset varies with the region stimulated and so does the length of sleep. One locus produced a sleep that generally lasted about 30 minutes, yet another produced sleep lasting as long as 4 hours. One locus produced a sleep so profound that the animal could not be awakened by noise or pinching, only by direct stimulation of the arousal system. In all of these instances the sleep included the natural EEG phases, both synchronous sleep and paradoxical sleep. This suggests that the subjective quality of sleep, the rapidity of onset, even the length of time we sleep, may be related to specific points along the hypnogenic path.

The term "pathway" suggests a narrow route, a roadway, differing from the terrain on either side.

This is an appropriate connotation, demonstrated by repeated experiments. After chemostimulating a particular site in an experimental animal, the researchers would wait for the cat to wake up and become fully alert. Then they moved the cannula a millimeter or two and repeated the stimulation. This time the chemical did not elicit sleep, but sometimes a very different kind of response. The acetylcholine that evoked sleep from one set of neurons aroused totally different activity within neurons not 1 millimeter away.

What has emerged from this extensive program of chemical brain mapping? Now, instead of islands of brain cells, inexplicably scattered, we see there is a whole pathway, shaped somewhat like a sickle, within the subcortical regions of the brain that produces sleep with cholinergic stimulation. It is connected, by fibers, with the cortex, that outer layer of cells involved in thought and the refinement of perception and emotion, from whence the voluntary commands to sleep may arise. It is connected with all the sensory modalities, and current exploration of the ascending pathway may explain how repetitious rhythms, like patting the cat, may put it to sleep. Depending upon where the circuit is touched, it produces sleep of different duration, profundity, and quality, which may help us to explain the different kinds of sleep we experience, out of boredom, after intense athletic exertion, following pleasant or wretched emotional experiences. A further finding may help to explain the restless sleep or insomnia that often occurs during periods of great worry.

During one study it was found that a spot evoking sleep with acetylcholine would produce an arousing effect if touched with noradrenalin. Other chemicals—GABA, adrenalin, nialimide—were tried but had no effect. Within this region the sleep path may come into close contact with the arousal system, perhaps overlapping or following the same route. Current experiments will explore this possibility by using noradrenalin as the stimulus. Once again there is the suggestion of a dual chemical code in which cholinergic compounds affect sleep-evoking cells and adrenergic compounds excite the cells of an antagonistic system—that of arousal (Cordeau, 1964).

The anatomical evidence for a relationship between sleep disorder and emotion does not yet explain insomnia, but it suggests some good topographical reasons why negative emotions might affect sleep.

"Motivation" and Sleep

Brain centers, colloquially known as "pleasure and pain" centers, have been located by electrical brain stimulation, beginning with the discovery of Dr. James Olds in the 1950's of a point in the hypothalamus that gave appearances of pleasure in the animals stimulated there. If motivation is determined by the "sense" of reward or punishment, or more neutrally, the positive or negative reinforcement that accompanies a behavior or thought, this center was indeed a motivation point. It appears to transmit impulses through fibers that pass through the medial forebrain bundle. The sleep system also transmits through this fiber bundle. This might suggest why pleasurable sensations often are accompanied by sleep. We might conceive that the positive motivational system is connected with neurons producing sleep. On the other hand, negative motivation seems to be connected with arousal, and indeed, a so-called "aversive" brain center, one producing negative feelings, has been located in a region that anatomically overlaps with the arousal center (Hernandez-Peon, in press).

These geographical findings do not explain insomnia, but they permit a hypothesis. When emotional excitement is intense, particularly when people worry, they cannot fall asleep easily. If this situation becomes prolonged, it may indicate that the arousal system is overactive, triggered into excitement by the emotional excitement in the limbic area nearby. There may be a very different explanation for the insomnia of some depressive and elderly people who cannot manage to stay asleep the whole night through. If some metabolic failure left the hypnogenic system without an adequate supply of acetylcholine, then it might run out of neural fuel, so to speak, and be unable to inhibit the arousal system for a full night. These are conjectural explanations at present, but they have considerable importance for therapy.

If we are to treat patients with insomnia or other sleep disorders to their greatest benefit, we must tailor drugs to the specific needs. These anatomical findings suggest means of testing drugs for their effects at particular loci in the brain. They may aid investigators who are now beginning to look at drug impact through evoked potentials and other neurophysiological and behavioral programs. Mappings of the sleep and arousal systems continue, and as we begin to acquire a more refined chart of systems within the brain and the chemical code that activates them, we have the prospect of developing specific remedies, offering needed sleep without hangovers, side-effects, depressions of mood, and without actually exaggerating the imbalances from which sleeplessness or disorder originated.

Chapter VI.
Control Over Sleep and
Other States of Consciousness

Singular feats of mental discipline and bodily control have marked certain individuals throughout history as almost superhuman. More admired than emulated, these incarnate gods have received their most rapturous worship from the ignorant or from children. They have been the yogi, calmly seated on bed of nails, or the Iroquois hero, silent and stoic during a savage beating, or the remarkable swami, standing on his head for hours at a time, inert as stone in contemplation. The commercial exploitation of these skills has led many adults to suspect that all fakirs indeed, must be fakes, for their performances seem beyond normal human attainment. When Rahman Bey spent 40 minutes at the bottom of the Hudson River in an air-tight coffin in the 1920's, Houdini followed suit in a debunking manner, inspiring Hamid Bey and others to a contest of live burials. But the secret was training. For centuries yogi have practised, under the name of pranayama, disciplines of restricted breathing among their many exercises, for which there are about 8½ million variations. The purpose is not a freakish prowess, but an integrated control of body and mind, allowing the individual full access to his consciousness.

Many eastern religions, among them Zen Buddhism, provide adherents with training in introspection and mental control, yet their goal of enlightened peace with the universe has seemed diffuse, appealing less to Westerners than combat tactics of jujitsu, karate, yogi acrobatics, or muscular relaxation procedures. These skills may seem more attainable than some of the supreme but subtle skills that have elevated our heroes. President Kennedy, for example, was being fitted for legend during his brief term of office, as people realized that he could ignore pain, command intense concentration, shifting focus at will, even sleeping at will. In the middle of a tense conference, as one White House consultant remembers, he called a break at a point of impasse and while others smoked or paced around, he leaned his head back and slept for a few minutes. Oddly enough, one of the more important contributions of sleep research in the long run may be that it can make these extraordinary mental disciplines available to all men. Research findings from the EEG laboratory have already indicated that it is possible to teach ordinary people control over a level of consciousness not usually experienced consciously. They have pointed to some of the unexplored phases of conscious states and the possibilities of utilizing them.

The ramifications are endless. If people could do something as simple as recognizing and describing the symptoms of illness, medical diagnosticians would be relieved of a time-consuming procedure—that of eliciting and then penetrating a confusing verbal cloud. The ability to fall asleep promptly, at will, has obvious merit. Moreover, recognition of the many tides of consciousness that continue in sleep and waking might allow people to seize their best moments, performing at the crest of their abilities. Most of us rise and fall on inner tides largely unaware and unable to recognize them, proceeding through life with only the barest acquaintanceship with our selves. Yoga literally means union. The body and mind are inseparable, and what we call mental discipline might permit a new approach in the treatment of medical, or psychosomatic disorders, and many forms of mental disorder. From extraordinary individuals we already know that voluntary control over pain, emotion, sleep, arousal, respiration, heart-rate, and many other functions must be possible.

Perhaps the biggest disadvantage to the curriculum of self-control in eastern religions is that it takes a long time, and the education does not begin in childhood. The posture of Zen meditation and shallow rhythmic breathing are difficult to learn, yet masters maintain this position for 7 and 8 hours. While meditating they may give every appearance of being asleep, yet they are in a state quite different from sleep. There is an anecdote about Dr. Baisetz Suzuki, a great Zen philosopher, as he attended a conference on Zen and Psychoanalysis. A guest of honor, he sat at a front table. He was then a man of 86, and during one particularly long session was thought to be asleep. He sat, immobile, eyes shut, unperturbed by events in the room, but when a breeze scuttled some papers down the table, it was Suzuki's hand that flashed out and secured them after they had passed the presumably alert participants at the head of the table. Suzuki had been in meditation, delicately balanced between relaxed detachment and instant alertness. This state is well known to electroencephalographers by its characteristic alpha rhythm.

Control of the Alpha Rhythm

Dr. Joe Kamiya, at Langley Porter Institute in San Francisco, has used the electroencephalograph as a teaching instrument demonstrating that control of the alpha state can be learned with surprising rapidity. Dr. Kamiya, in previous studies of sleep and dreaming, was struck with the difficulty professed by volunteers in communicating their dreams and other subjective experiences. However honest a person may be, most people are notoriously inept at describing subjective events. For this reason, many studies of perception, pain, and sleep have sidestepped introspective accounts. Indeed, modern psychology has shunned introspection. As a result we know little about the manner in which civilized people acquire self-control, how they exercise mental discipline and begin to recognize and communicate their feelings.

An infant can do nothing more than cry when something hurts. The child, after some coaxing from his parents, may point to his stomach. He learns to say that his stomach hurts, and eventually he may discriminate between a stabbing pain and an ache. He will be almost mature before he can describe his emotions even crudely. His discrimination between inmost levels of consciousness will probably remain aboriginal. The rich qualitative variation between deep sleep and high arousal does not even have a vocabulary. For example, most people experience the alpha state many times each day, but they would not know how to identify it.

The characteristic alpha rhythm of about 9–12 c.p.s. appears when a person relaxes with eyes closed. This isn't drowsiness. The rhythm vanishes on the threshold of sleep and also when a person becomes tense, emotionally upset, or gripped by a problem. A Japanese EEG study of Zen Buddhist monks has reportedly shown that the meditation state is a sustained period of alpha rhythm. Sustaining this rhythm is no mean trick, for any call to attention, sudden thought, or outside distraction disrupts it. A study of the alpha state was a logical first step in exploring the process of introspection because it occurs during wakefulness and is easily identified on the EEG.

Six years ago Dr. Kamiya and his associates wondered whether a native volunteer could be taught to identify the occurrence of his alpha rhythm. They placed electrodes on a volunteer's head, bade him lie down in an experimental bedroom and told him that a bell would occasionally ring, sometimes when alpha waves appeared, sometimes during other EEG patterns. He was asked to guess whether or not the bell had rung during alpha and was told whether he was right or wrong. By the fourth session the volunteer was always correct in his guess and discriminated correctly 400 times in a row. Six other volunteers achieved 70–100 percent accuracy on 50–500 trials. Surely it looked as if they had learned to use some internal cues to identify an inner experience they had never known before. But there was a remote chance that the bell sounded different during alpha than nonalpha, and the procedure was varied to obviate this possibility.

Now the volunteers were instructed to say "yes" when they felt they were in alpha and "no" when they weren't. This, too, they did with great accuracy. A number of physiological measures were taken—heart rate, respiration, eye movements, and muscle tension— to see whether one of these changed during alpha, providing the cue. Although previous studies never indicated a relationship between alpha and heart or respiration changes, this precautionary check gave evidence that ruled out palpitation of the heart, a change in muscle tension, respiration, and eye movements as cues.

The initial volunteer, the experimenters had noticed, had inadvertently learned to control his alpha rhythm once he learned to identify it. Volunteers in a subsequent study were told to induce alpha or suppress it on command, giving an alpha rhythm when a single tone sounded and eliminating it when two tones sounded. None of the volunteers knew the name of the state they were trying to manipulate. They knew that a "yes" was associated with one sensation and a "no" with another. When the tone sounded once, the volunteer conjured up the "yes" state. As they watched the EEG record in the control room, the experimenters were amazed to see an alpha rhythm appear after a single tone and vanish after the double tone.

The next variation of the experiment required a technical innovation. An electrical filter, calibrated to pass only the subject's dominant alpha rhythm, would sound a tone. Now the tone was automatically controlled by the subject's alpha rhythm; in a sense, his very thought controlled the tone. The tone started whenever alpha appeared and stayed on until the alpha vanished. Subjects were told to keep that tone off. They were to suppress alpha. These volunteers were new to the study. They had never learned to identify alpha, nevertheless they were able to keep the tone from sounding most of the time. How had they learned to control a subtle mental state for which they had no name?

When they were asked, the volunteers said that the alpha state was serene, pleasant, and devoid of visual imagery. Some volunteers said they "saw" things in order to suppress alpha, and these visions were often floating spots, faces, headlines. Then the tone went off. It took some effort to keep the tone silent, they said, for when they maintained alpha on command they found they could forget about outside stimulation—including the tone. Not all of the volunteers were equally adept, but the first eight subjects became skilled at turning alpha on and off. When it was on, they said, they were relaxed yet vigilant—like Dr. Suzuki?

The pleasant alpha suspension was quickly banished when they exerted mental effort, evoked images, or tried to solve a problem. When asked to maintain alpha and add memorized figures, the subject either maintained alpha and did incorrect arithmetic, or he did correct arithemtic and lost alpha. Some people in other studies have managed to solve simple problems and maintain alpha, and it has been speculated that it depends upon the amount of visualization employed.

Zen teaching is based upon the awakening of inner perception to the core of one's being by an inward listening that is destroyed by logic or effort of intellect. One student of Zen has described the sustained meditation as a portal to a poetic illumination, an appreciation of all physical self and nature—resembling the paradise of a child and incompatible with objective thinking. A student of Zen may learn to sustain meditation, after many years, and to achieve the state known as enlightenment—perhaps what might be described as a union with the unconscious. Dr. Kamiya's laboratory is attempting to see how long the alpha state can be held by volunteers with a few hours of practice. This study may explain one of the perplexing and repeated facts of history—that monks and moguls have been said to meditate continuously for many hours a day and to do with little sleep. Participants in a Zen retreat sometimes meditate for as long as 17 hours at a stretch and have been known to go without sleep for 5 days or more. Recently, one participant in a retreat, a Chicago housewife, is reported to have meditated for 5 days without sleep. According to Dr. Albert

J. Stunkard of the University of Pennsylvania, she showed no signs of fatigue. When introduced into a conventional social situation she acted with her accustomed propriety and responsiveness and suffered no distortions of vision, time, or other effects usually associated with prolonged sleep loss.

Voluntary Control and Psychosomatic Medicine

Further EEG and polygraph studies may reveal whether the alpha state does indeed perform some of the functions of sleep and what its special physiological properties may be. By using the EEG in a feedback system for instruction, Dr. Kamiya has been able to train people to identify, control, and sustain a state in a manner that apparently takes years to achieve by Zen training. The same procedure will be used in attempts to instruct people in the control of other EEG patterns that correlate with mental states. If, indeed, the EEG picture corresponds with mental events this research adventure is opening up the possibility of internal education, avenues of instruction in mental control. People may, indeed, learn to discriminate between the stages of sleep (Antrobus, 1965) and learn how to awaken during a particular phase, as some people do awaken at a regular time without aid from alarm clocks. How does one "conquer" pain, "subdue" anger, reduce one's breathing, stop one's heart?

We are now acquiring the tools to explore some of the "superhuman" feats of the past. Simulated death, for instance, and heart stoppage were the trick of a famous prisoner in an American prison who used to astound the doctors by lying down—dead—then returning to life. This apparent inhibition of sympathetic-autonomic activity resembles the occurrences in the process of falling asleep and is an integral part of yogi meditation. At one time investigators reported that an accomplished yogi could suspend his heart beat for 18 seconds. The observations were made by taking the pulse and listening, but electrocardiograms have shown that the heart doesn't stop. Instead, the volume of each beat is so diminished that only a most sensitive instrument will detect it. How was this imperceptible volume attained? Surely reduced heart beat is not accomplished as directly as moving an arm, although one step may be under direct voluntary control. By expanding the lungs one can put pressure on the heart and reduce its volume. The yogi feat takes skill and practice, but it resembles something that anyone can try for himself. One can produce an increased heart rate very simply by thinking alarming thoughts or conjuring up fearsome memories. Current findings by Dr. Kamiya also suggest that blood pressure can be conditioned downward.

The autonomic nervous system, the involuntary system that controls heart rate, perspiration, and many vital functions, is now believed to play an active role in many psychosomatic diseases: heart ailments, ulcers, colitis, headaches, and skin diseases. If people can learn to control their mental and emotional forces, they will also be controlling many of their physiological functions. Such a development might put us on the road toward teaching patients to diminish their own symptoms and also to prevent psychosomatic disease, providing a very interesting technique, moreover, to the psychotherapist. Research into the way we develop our introspective faculties, by offering us tools for further education, could have a profound value well beyond practical possibilities for medicine and psychiatry. Such an education could surely, to use the succinct cliché, enrich the lives of people now compressed from every side by an overpopulous, overregulated, and increasingly technical society. The Utopian goal of inward cultivation is more distant, however, than some of the more limited forms of control we may be able to acquire.

Sleep Learning

Sleep learning has been a particularly intriguing possibility. If we could learn French or electrical engineering during sleep, practical advantages are manifold. Could we take courses during sleep? Could our lives be enriched by other kinds of useful training during sleep? Could our sleeping lives provide a part of our total education, a part of character formation, or even therapy? During the last 20 years there has been a welter of conflicting evidence, and these questions are by no means settled. Recent studies in Russia (Kulikov, 1964) and the United States (Evans et al., 1965; Cobb et al., 1964) suggest that it is possible for hypnotic subjects to understand relatively complicated things during sleep. Indeed, it has been said that the Russians have succeeded in teaching some English during sleep, but most American scientists remain skeptical.

Studies of sleep behavior and neurophysiology have begun to map out some of the limits and possibilities of sleep learning and to illumine how the sleeping brain reacts and what it is capable of doing. Many people, of course, assume that sleep teaching is a reliable if slightly miraculous commercial technique offering success in acquiring skills without effort. The great commercial endeavor began around 1947 when a successful distributor of foreign language records began selling the records with a loudspeaker designed to be placed under the pillow and a phonograph that turned on and off automatically. Advertisements said that this equipment would enable people to learn a language during sleep. By 1958 the business had so expanded that there were records to improve salesmanship, to break habits, to enforce diets, to enable a person to become financially successful—a more than $10 million business.

During the mid-1950's Dr. Charles W. Simon and William Emmons at the Rand Corp. took a close look at the sleep-learning literature which then included a spate of scientific studies, some of them weakly supporting the claim that instruction in sleep improved waking performance. Simon and Emmons ran their own EEG study and decided that if they saw alpha rhythm in the record they would not assume the subject was asleep. Even with volunteers of high intelligence, there was no evidence that material "stuck" if presented during slow-wave sleep, and signs of learning diminished as alpha diminished. They concluded that there was no good case for factual learning during sleep, although some other form of training might be possible, perhaps the use of drowsy states to modify attitudes and supplement waking training or psychotherapy. They suggested an exploration of the many waking states of consciousness that are far beneath an optimum alertness.

The Simon and Emmons papers performed a cleansing within the murky realm of sleep learning. They did not, however, debunk the issue. If factual learning of repeated words did not seem to occur in sleep, this did not mean that records playing throughout the night failed to penetrate the brain or that they might not have some effect during the alpha state before sleep.

Subsequent behavioral and neurophysiological researches have amplified the case against a straightforward sleep teaching—presented as a progression of facts. The different sleep phases have different properties, first of all. As Webb and others have shown, slow-wave sleep occupies a goodly proportion of the initial part of the night. Slow-wave sleep would appear to be the least amenable for conventional teaching. In a number of experiments demonstrating that people can make responses such as pressing a button during sleep, the responses more rarely occurred during slow-wave sleep of stages 3 and 4. Quite a number of investigators have charted the brain's EEG response to a stimulus during sleep, and these studies of evoked potentials may help to explain the apparent impermeability of this phase of sleep.

In recent studies, Rosner and his associates at the West Haven, Conn., Veterans Administration Hospital compared the waking and sleeping brain responses of people who were repeatedly given a mild electric shock, causing a slight tingle at the median nerve of the wrist. Analyses of the EEG responses from many people and many nights corroborated the many data that REM sleep bears a close resemblance to waking but that slow-wave sleep is quite different. Using sounds as stimuli in a study at Walter Reed, Williams found that people gave EEG responses that changed in shape in the various stages of sleep much like the responses to wrist shock (Williams et al., 1962, 1963). Using quite another method, Dr. W. R. Adey and his laboratory at UCLA have detected shifts in impedance, the electrical resistance of neural tissue at deep brain sites during sleep and waking. Drs. David Foulkes in Chicago and Joe Kamiya in San Francisco have found that people report different kinds of mentation in slow-wave sleep than in REM sleep, generally remembering far less. Now, the findings of Dr. Rosner and his associates suggest why mentation during slow-wave sleep may be vastly different from that of waking or the REM phase of intense dreaming.

Projecting in all directions from the thalamus are small nerve fibers that finally refer sensory information to the entire cortex, a diffuse projection system that is thought to be essential to conscious awareness. Brain wave patterns, inferred to emanate from this region, appear toward the end of the EEG response to a stimulus. They do not disappear in sleep, but arrive later and progressively larger as sleep moves from stage 1 to stage 4. It would seem that it takes longer for the integrative process to begin in this deep sleep, showing what might be called a slower reaction time, and longer for the process to occur. This suggests a kind of slow motion in mental activity. Since speed of function plays a role in the quality of thought, this evidence suggests that REM mentation would more nearly resemble that of waking. During slow-wave sleep, moreover, the latter part of the EEG response showed a shape that was the reverse of the waking equivalent. A negative wave occurred where a positive existed in waking. The meaning of all this is not known in detail, but it certainly adds to the evidence that says the brain's function is far different in slow-wave sleep than waking. One might not expect success in teaching by methods that are timed for a waking brain.

Roughly one-fifth of the night and a goodly portion of the later part of the night is spent in a phase of sleep that, by all the accumulated data, seems closest to waking: stage 1 REM. The shape of the EEG response to stimulation is closest to the waking response in this period. This is the time of vivid dreaming and a great variety of behaviors, perhaps a time when specially timed teaching procedures might prove effective. Obtaining responses from people in this stage of sleep is not like asking a waking person to do something, however, and the particular properties of this sleep stage can be glimpsed in some of the recent research.

Discriminations During Sleep

At a time when sleep learning looked like a dead issue, two laboratories, separated by a continent, were quietly at work reopening the possibility. Kamiya and his associates at Langley Porter in San Francisco were offering their volunteers money as a reward for performing during sleep. The performance was not complicated. When a tone sounded, they were to press a thumb switch. Because the tone had been coupled to the onset of the REM period, the investigators wondered whether subjects would begin to associate rapid eye movements with the tone without awakening. Many people felt that motivation was important, and Kamiya's subjects began to act as if they were learning the relationship of tone and REMs—especially when the money payments increased. After about 4 hours they were pressing the thumb switch just a little before the eye movements began. This suggested that they had associated the tone with the eye movements and had learned internal sensations perhaps "warning" them that the eye movement period was about to begin. They were able, therefore, to tell the outside world that they were dreaming or were about to dream.

A subject in a New York laboratory also learned to discriminate between the REM state and other sleep (Antrobus et al., 1964). How does a sleeping person tell the difference between one phase of sleep and another? Does his inner experience in some way reflect changes that correspond with the marked changes observed on the EEG record? Does he detect unusual body movement, respiration, eye motions, vivid dreams? In pursuing this problem, Dr. Antrobus has not asked subjects to press a switch during a particular stage of sleep, but has asked for verbal identification upon awakenings. Can a person learn to identify different stages of sleep as he can learn to identify alpha rhythm? A study of one woman strongly suggests that a person can learn to discriminate about his inner sleeping experience (Antrobus, 1965). The nurse in this study was awakened during REM sleep and stage 2. Although she knew them only as "A" or "B," she was asked to guess in which phase she had been prior to awakening and was always told whether or not she was correct. This training procedure lasted some 16 nights, and by the last 4 nights the subject was almost 100 percent correct. Asked how she discriminated, she said she felt that there was something in the quality of the sleep, the quality of the dreaming, and the depth of sleep.

Now the experimenter wanted to find out whether rapid eye movements provided a cue. On several nights the subject was awakened during REM periods only during intervals when the eyes were not moving, and also during stage 2 sleep. Once again, the subject was nearly perfect in her discrimination and so it did not appear that rapid eye movements themselves dictated her correct discrimination of the REM stage.

A further step, requiring the discrimination of still another phase of sleep has not been conclusive. However, it does seem that the subjective quality of REM sleep and stage 2 permit a person to distinguish between them. Individuals vary in their sensitivity to internal experience, and most people are inarticulate about subjective events, so that it may take considerable exploration of this kind before there is a verbal map even crudely describing the "feeling" of the EEG stages of sleep. It is perhaps ironic that the experimenters and their cooperative subjects now haltingly trying to describe how they distinguish between the EEG stages of sleep are mapping a territory less known than the space traversed by the astronauts, uncharted seas of consciousness through which we all pass unknowingly every night of our lives.

Performance During Sleep

It has been clear in diverse studies of sleep behavior that people differ considerably in their reactions and their sensitivities. In addition, the techniques of study have varied considerably. In one study of sleep discrimination the volunteers were motivated to perform in sleep by punishment for failure to respond. At the beginning of each REM period a light went on, as a cue to the sleeping person that he was about to enter a REM period. If he did not respond within a minute, a buzzer sounded. When he pressed a switch 10 times, the light went off. There are a number of variations of this experiment, and in one series subjects were mildly shocked if they failed to press the switch. Some subjects apparently needed little coaxing, and their performance would improve from night to night without punishment, while some people apparently got used to lights, buzzers, shocks, and showed little inclination to perform (Hammack, 1962–64). Subjects in another laboratory were receiving even stronger inducements to perform in the form of what might seem even more irritating punishment for failure.

In the studies of Dr. Harold L. Williams and his associates at Walter Reed, the volunteers slept with a microswitch taped in their right hands, and they were told to close it whenever a tone sounded. They were given three nights of grace. For these first nights there were no dire consequences if they failed to close the switch when the tone sounded, and the tone was automatically turned off. However, life was different on the next three nights. Now if the subject failed to close the microswitch within 4 seconds of the tone, a fire alarm began ringing, lights flashed, and his leg was shocked. Two of the subjects had been asked to discriminate between an irrelevant and a critical tone. If they ignored the irrelevant tone nothing happened, but failure to close the switch after the critical tone brought on the noise, flashing lights, and shock.

The motivating power of punishment was clearly important. On the nights of grace with no punishment for failure, the subjects hardly responded, almost not at all during REM sleep. On the nights when failure meant punishment, however, they were responding to the critical tone during all phases of sleep. The biggest improvement could be seen in the REM period, and one subject responded 85 percent of the time when the critical tone was played during REM sleep (Williams et al., 1963, 1964).

Memory

These studies suggested that some kind of learning might occur during sleep, that people indeed might be taught to discriminate between the phases of sleep. They emphasized the importance of motivation in getting anybody to do anything during sleep. A further aspect of sleep performance was emphasized by a study at UCLA.

Drs. Mary and Arnold Mandell and Allen Jacobson used encouragement and careful instruction before sleep to motivate their subjects. The volunteers were told that they would hear numbers during their sleep. The task was to listen to the spoken numbers and remember them but not to wake up until the experimenter invited waking. The recorded numbers were played and after 10 seconds the volunteer was awakened. If the numbers were played during slow-wave sleep the volunteers claimed they never heard them. However, they were able to recite the numbers played during REM sleep and reported that the numbers sometimes entered a dream (Mandell et al., 1965). Ten seconds, however, is a very short time. Further experiments are exploring the limits of memory during sleep.

One of these studies has simply involved awakening the subject during sleep, presenting a word, and varying the amount of time the person remains awake before falling back asleep. In the morning the volunteers have been given tests of recall and recognition for the words they had seen and pronounced during the night. Retention, it would seem, depends upon how soon the person receiving the word goes back to sleep. If permitted to fall asleep almost directly, he appears to forget—suggesting that sleep, itself, can prevent the forming of a memory (Portnoff et al., 1965).

The shortness of memory for sleep events may account for one's ability to get up in the morning and feel that the night was spent in an oblivion as deep as death. The last few years of research has certainly shown that, far from being dead asleep, the sleeping person is mentally active, capable of behaviors of many varieties—talking, walking, dreaming, thinking, and he is impressively sensitive to significant events. This discrimination, which as Ian Orwald demonstrated, permits a person to sleep through a stream of names but awaken to the sound of his own name, is a most impressive daily occurrence, yet one we take quite for granted. It is expressed as "the baby's cry phenomenon" by many investigators. A mother may sleep through a violent thunderstorm yet awaken if her baby coughs or cries (Oswald, 1960, 1961, 1962).

Experiments in Discrimination

People don't stop to marvel at the fact that they can sleep through familiar noises yet waken if the baby cries or a burglarlike footfall occurs in the house. Dr. Jose P. Segundo and his associates at UCLA have undertaken an experimental analysis of this important discrimination. Their subjects were cats implanted with electrodes. While awake, they were trained to discriminate between several tones that were close together in pitch so that one of the tones became associated with a shock to the paw. First, however, they heard all tones over and over again until they simply did not react when they heard any of them. Then the critical tone was paired with shock. However, if the cat responded to the tone by meaowing or flexing its paw, it managed to avoid the shock. The whole gamut of other tones were played, meanwhile, without shock. Now the animal was tested during sleep.

During all phases of sleep, the cats discriminated between the critical tone and the irrelevant ones. This was apparent on the EEG and in behavior. Whenever the critical tone sounded, the EEG patterns shifted toward the characteristic fast rhythms of arousal. This happened before the cats even moved. However, when the irrelevant tones sounded, there was no such arousal, or at least it was far less frequent. These cats had not learned during sleep, but applied during sleep learning acquired during wakefulness, as in the manner of people sleeping through traffic sounds but alerting to the opening of a door.

The investigators subsequently pursued the possibility of sleep learning. Implanted cats, fast asleep, were shocked lightly when a certain tone was sounded. To avoid shock they merely had to alert themselves, and an EEG arousal pattern permitted them to escape punishment. The training procedure was particularly delicate, as might be imagined. Only a few shocks could be delivered during any one session or the cat might become too upset to sleep. However, it was soon clear that the cats did learn to associate the tone and the shock, and the tone elicited the EEG picture of arousal. Strictly speaking, this may not have been sleep learning, because the training shocks had awakened them. The association of the tone with the subsequent shocks probably occurred after the shocks arrived and therefore in a wakeful animal. The shock was then associated with the memory of the tone heard in sleep (Segundo, 1964; Buendia et al., 1963).

The issue of memory span during sleep was underscored by these studies. During sleep, the trace following the tone—a brain wave pattern whose duration may indicate memory span for the signal—is far smaller than during waking. Dr. Segundo and his associates varied the interval between tone and shock, and found that if it were too long the animal never seemed to learn the relation. A tone, followed by shock within 16 seconds, for instance, was apparently connected by the sleeping animal, and it learned to alert to the tone. However, when the shock followed the tone after 32 seconds, the sleeping animal apparently never connected the two events and never learned to avoid shock (Izquierdo et al.).

Material designed for learning in sleep apparently requires special pacing. It would seem that relationships can be imparted by presenting the related items—whether they are words or something else—close together in time.

In a human study somewhat analogous to the cat study, subjects discriminated between a significant (shock-paired) tone and a neutral tone by showing a particular brain wave formation whenever the meaningful tone was played during deep sleep (Beh and Barratt, 1965). These subjects who had been given chloral hydrate to induce sleep showed no signs of shifting into a lighter stage of sleep. Tests given to the subjects later, during waking, showed that the significance that had been conditioned during sleep carried over into the waking state. The importance of this recent work is precisely that sleep-conditioning did not arouse the subject and that it did carry over into waking. This study underscores one of the most mysterious aspects of recent studies of sleep learning and memory.

Many investigators have emphasized the individual differences they have observed and the by no means uniform success in sleep-conditioning. Some people awaken. Others do not respond. When asked to recall dreams or words heard during sleep, people have displayed a readiness to forget rather than remember. In general, these results dampened the hope of accomplishing very much by sleep training, and surely the unsophisticated attempts and commercial programs of the past had not been encouraging. There is, however, a singular group of people who seem to react differently to sleep instruction and display faculties of memory for sleep learning. Nobody has determined what properties of mind distinguished these people, only that they are capable of being hypnotized.

Sleep Learning in Hypnotic Subjects

A recent Russian study of sleep instruction was performed on schoolchildren who had shown signs of suggestibility. After the children were asleep for an hour or two, a tape recorder was turned on at subthreshold levels. The child was told to continue sleeping deeply and to listen and remember the text. The recorded text was either a Tolstoy story, or, if the child had shown some interest in Pavlovian psychology, the text contained material on higher nervous activity. When the text had been played, the subject was told to remember it forever and to sleep on. When tested on this material during waking, a good many of the subjects could repeat the text without knowing how they had learned the material and performed as well as children who had been given the material during waking (Kulikov, 1964). There are a good many questions to be asked about the way in which this study was run. So many investigators have failed to inculcate even simple material during sleep that this report may arouse some skepticism. However, a team of investigators at the Institute of Pennsylvania Hospital have elicited an equally startling, and perhaps related, response in hypnotizable adults.

This study was undertaken in order to find out whether responsiveness to suggestion during sleep would permit hypnosis in a person of low suggestibility. Eight young men participated in the study, four of them demonstrably of high suggestibility, four of them unresponsive. The procedure was simple. The volunteer wore EEG electrodes and went to sleep in the laboratory bedroom naturally, without hypnotic suggestion. During stage 1 sleep he was instructed to move his pillow whenever he heard the word "pillow," and during the deeper stages of sleep he heard an instruction to scratch his nose whenever he heard the word "itch." The four deeply hypnotizable subjects responded very differently from the less suggestible subjects who either gave no response or showed signs of waking. The deeply hypnotizable subjects, on the contrary, followed instruction whenever it was administered in stage 1 sleep. Although they would scratch noses and move pillows at the mention of the cue word, they did not recall any of this when awakened in the morning.

The results have been replicated using a larger sample of 20 subjects who had not previously been screened for susceptibility to hypnosis. In the course of a free association test the next day, they did react to cue words that were slipped in. More striking than that sign of carryover, however, was their performance on the subsequent night. Presented with cue words on a second night, without any repetition of the instructions, they responded again in sleep. When subsequently tested for susceptibility to hypnosis, a significant but low correlation was obtained between susceptibility to hypnosis and the rate of responding to the sleep suggestion (Cobb et al., 1964; Cobb et al., 1965; Evans et al., 1965).

Why does the deeply suggestible person follow instructions in sleep? What mysterious mental attributes allow him not only to receive instruction during sleep but to respond during waking and subsequent sleep? Studies of hypnotic subjects may help to reveal overlooked possibilities in sleep learning. Efforts to find out what suggestibility means, and something about the hypnotic subject's memory process, may also indicate whether elaborate sleep learning can be accomplished in the ordinary person. During a recent pilot study at the University of Pennsylvania, Drs. J. P. Brady and B. S. Rosner found that the hypnotic suggestion to dream produces a trance state with a waking brain wave pattern accompanied by the rapid eye movements that are characteristic of the vivid dreaming phase. Dreams reported by these hypnotic subjects sounded almost indistinguishable from nightly dreams, but unlike nighttime dreams that seem to evaporate from memory within seconds, these hypnotic dreams have been remembered

10 minutes and longer in great detail.

It is interesting that only the hypnotizable subjects showed rapid eye movements during their dreams. Other subjects were able to manufacture dreams but had no conjugate eye movements. Was the hypnotized dreamer able to "switch on" part of the brain activity involved in nightly dreaming? Is the suggestible person capable of using his brain, manipulating his state of consciousness, differently than the normal person? Can he voluntarily "turn on" brain states that we customarily think of as involuntary? EEG studies like this one may eventually begin to characterize the way in which the hypnotizable person functions by elucidating the brain activity in persons who seem especially receptive to instruction and capable of retention. If it is possible to discover how the suggestible person uses his brain or, indeed, what brain mechanisms are called into play in acceding to a hypnotic suggestion, it may also be possible to teach such internal manipulations to "non-suggestible" persons. Such a possibility might open the door to unforeseen advances in psychotherapy. If elaborate sleep learning does indeed occur and depends upon suggestibility, a greater understanding of the nature of hypnosis may make such sleep learning techniques available and useful to humanity. This knowledge is likely to take a long time in the gathering and will probably attract attention long before the evidence is obtained, because it is one of the more glamorous aspects of the problem—the yet unanswered question—of learning complicated material during sleep. A good deal of our insight may come from neurophysiological studies where already, in far less sensational facets of sleep learning, we have observed one aspect that is exhibited by all normal people and animals.

Habituation

One kind of learning that does seem to occur during sleep—as it does during waking—is negative learning. We rapidly learn not to get alarmed about meaningless events. With cats, if the critical tone were repeated without shock, the tone soon produced no arousal response, and the creature slept through the night. This kind of extinction permits a person to adjust to a noisy neighborhood or to sleep on a train or plane. The learning by which one does react to meaningful events, remaining unreactive to trivia, is essential for survival, and for each individual it is somewhat different, since each life follows a singular course. What kind of brain mechanism would give us this power of discrimination?

Segundo and his associates conjectured that the learned response is mediated by a neural "receptor stage" that detects and identifies the outside event. This discharges a "trigger mechanism" according to pitch or intensity. Finally, an "affector mechanism" would organize the conditioned response. In tracking this mechanism to its very brain cells, the next study utilized microelectrodes implanted within single cells in the mesencephalic reticular formation in cats. This is the region that participates in arousing the animal. Here, perhaps, one might see how the critical stimulus finally elicited arousal in the animal.

This was an elaborate study, but briefly it involved stimulating the cat—perhaps by a touch on the shoulder, or by speaking to it, or turning up the light in the room—and cataloging the discharge of the implanted neurons. Relative to the number of cells in this region very few were surveyed, yet the survey showed cellular activity in unbelievable variety. Different cells responded to different sense signals—some handling several, others only reacting to one. Some cells discharged regularly, like a metronome, regardless of stimulation. Others responded in a restricted manner only when stimulation was applied in the form of a touch to the right upper lip, for instance, or the hairs of the cheek. Some fired almost instantly, others after a long delay. The diversity of function and mode of function was enormous (Bell et al., 1964).

When a nerve cell is repeatedly stimulated it begins to discharge less. However, cells attenuated differently. Some adapted to sound faster than light but if allowed a rest would discharge when restimulated. Some cells appeared particularly sensitive to novelty, quickly attenuating in their response after repeated stimulation. In this array of receptor cells, novelty and habituation to sensory stimulation were richly represented—providing a means of conveying "significance." This may be the neural background of a most important kind of learning, for an obvious survival value attaches to the ability to sleep through the irrelevant yet awaken when external events are meaningful or threatening. By what code did the cells convey their messages to a trigger mechanism in the next step toward a response? Neural messages resemble a code of pulses and spaces rhythmically organized—a kind of Morse code composed only of dots and pauses in tempo. In a further study of a single giant nerve cell within a mollusk, Segundo and his associates are attempting to learn something about this code (Moore et al., 1963; Segundo et al., 1963).

The learning involved in controlling sleep onset has not yet been explicated in quite the same manner. We all know that some people can fall asleep almost instantly at will, but how they do it remains a mystery. They may be particularly sensitive to body cues. Perhaps they pick the right moment to decide to fall asleep so that the element of "will power" is combined with sensitive adjustment to internal rhythms and some training. As fairly recent studies have demonstrated, it is possible to condition sleep in a classical manner. Pavlov used morphine injection to condition sleep in dogs for whom the preliminaries of injection were cues to fall asleep. His more famous dogs salivated at the sound of a bell, but the cats and monkeys of a current UCLA experiment fall asleep.

Conditioning Sleep

Drs. Carmine D. Clemente and M. B. Sterman at UCLA were probably the first to condition implanted cats to fall asleep at the sound of a tone (Clemente et al., 1963). A survey of the literature led them to expect that stimulation in an area in the basal forebrain might cause synchronous waves, the waves of sleep, to emanate from

184

the cortex. Using an electrode in what is now known as the forebrain synchronizing area, they would stimulate a cat, and it would drop into sleep in 1–2 minutes. Through a window in each cage, the implanted cats could be watched as they wandered around. They would receive a stimulation, and the EEG record would change from the low-voltage waking script to the rolling waves of sleep. The animal would lie down and close its eyes. Altering the voltage and the length of stimulation had pronounced effect. At a voltage just over 1.5 volts, a cat who had just assumed a death grip on a live rat would, in the moment of throttling, drop the rat and retreat drowsily to a corner and sleep.

The cats did not seem to mind this stimulation at all. They willingly entered the recording cages. Some of them purred. Once they had adjusted to stimulation, a neutral tone was added. The tone was sounded with the stimulation. After many pairings, the tone, by itself, was enough to make the cat sleepy and produce the EEG signs of sleep.

An analogous experiment has been performed by Drs. Clemente and Knauss on monkeys whose reactions are closer to man's. This classical conditioning may explain why many of us fall asleep at a habitual time, even though we are not particularly tired. We have many habits surrounding sleep, rituals of washing, turning out lights, and associated cues including bedrooms, bedclothes, etc. This routine is conditioned in childhood and much of it persists throughout life. Perhaps radically different habits could be trained in infancy. Dr.

Clemente has speculated that we might learn to sleep less. One way to explore the possibility is to condition very young animals to sleep less than they normally would. The first step in such studies is a collection of data indicating how much a certain species does, indeed, sleep. Normative data on cats shows that they appear to be drowsy 15 percent of the time, spend 40 percent of the time in slow-wave sleep, and about a third of the time awake, the remainder in paradoxical sleep (Sterman et al., 1964).

Stimulation of the forebrain synchronizing area, coupled with a tone that permitted conditioning, suggested that this brain region might be implicated in habit formation and sleep regulation. After the normative study of cat sleep, each animal was given a surgical lesion, knocking out large numbers of nerve cells in the forebrain synchronizing area. After this surgery the cats slept less and drowsed less. Further study of this brain area may tell us a great deal about hypnotic trance, coma, anesthesia, and the way in which voluntary or conditioned controls evolve. The basal forebrain contains a reinforcing center or "pleasure center" that may well be involved in the forming of habits.

Sleep Habits

Habit, no doubt, plays some role in falling asleep at night. Indeed, many people who take daytime naps will perform part of their nightly ritual, undressing and climbing into bed in order to sleep, in accordance with the famous prescription of Sir Winston Churchill who felt that this was the way to obtain a refreshing nap. When and how are these sleep habits formed? Does infant training exert a lifelong influence? A good deal of information has emerged from the studies of Dr. Wilse B. Webb and his associates at Gainesville, Fla. (Webb, 1957–65; Agnew et al., 1964; Williams et al., 1964).

In a look at family sleeping habits, a questionnaire survey has been conducted among 600 people whose ages range from 8 years to 80. This large group includes people who were reared according to two very different infant feeding fads. Some had been awakened on schedule for feeding during infancy while others were fed on demand. Insofar as the questionnaire could indicate, there was no clear relationship between these very different experiences in infancy and later sleep habits. Animal studies have been showing that the younger the animal the more flexible is his sleep response. Young rats can maintain themselves for long periods on a constantly rotating water wheel by sleeping in 10–15 second bursts, whereas older rats much more quickly fatigue and fall off the wheel. Questionnaire responses have shown that the amount of time a person sleeps is related to his age, the lifetime pattern forming a U-shaped curve in which infants and the elderly sleep the most. The number of times a person awakens during the night is also related to age and increases with age. In all age groups, however, there seemed to be a very striking and consistent relationship between "good" sleep and what our grandmothers might have prescribed as "regular sleep habits." People who maintained a regular bedtime and regular time of awakening generally reported that it was easy to go to sleep, suffered fewer nighttime awakenings, and felt refreshed when they awakened in the morning.

There may be some relationship between this finding and recent evidence from the animal laboratory. Using rats as subjects, this laboratory has investigated many factors that might alter the likelihood of falling asleep. For instance, it has been found that sound might cause an animal to take a long time falling asleep whereas light had no such effect. Rats are diurnal animals. Normally, they sleep during the daytime. Although rats vary as individuals, some falling asleep with ease, others showing a tendency to have difficulty in falling asleep, the most significant determinant of their sleep response appears to be the diurnal periodicity. External means of encouraging them to fall asleep rapidly are far more effective during the daytime, during their normal sleep period, than at night when the rat would normally be awake. Although little is known about the metabolic clocks within the body that may produce this periodicity, they normally appear to be quite regular. Perhaps the maintenance of a regular bed time enables people to take advantage of such periodicities within their bodies.

Sleeping habits employ external cues such as turning out lights, but they also involve internal cues, thoughts, and emotions. Advice on falling asleep usually contains the admonition: "Think of pleasant things." If that fails, bore yourself to sleep with a repetitive sequence—counting sheep. Counting sheep, or being rocked in a cradle are repetitive stimuli that may be related to the direct electrical stimulation that causes animals to sleep. It is interesting to note that the stimulation, by which Dr. Clemente and his associates obtained sleep in cats, was of low frequency. The frequency was similar to that of the synchronized waves of sleep. We may yet discover that a rhythmic event, timed like that of a person's sleep brain waves, is indeed soporific.

Voluntary control over sleep may, in addition, require more sensitivity to internal body cues than most of us learn in our lives. If cycles of physiological change and mental states indicate an optimum time for falling asleep, we might learn to heed our fluctuations in attention, sense of heat or chill, muscular coordination, and other cues. A number of studies on the determinants of sleep may reveal whether we do, indeed, ignore such cues and whether there are optimum periods for falling asleep.

The Awakening Process

It is also conceivable that people may learn from current sleep studies useful information about the process of awakening and when awakening occurs most easily. Until recently there has been little interest in the process of awakening. Studies in the Gainesville, Fla., laboratory have indicated that people show great individual differences even when their motivation, training, and tasks are constant. Measurements of handgrip, for instance, suggest that muscular strength may be low when a person first awakens, returning slowly to the normal waking level (Webb and Jeanneret; Webb and Agnew). More recent work suggests that an important factor in the ease of awakening is not the length of time a person has been asleep but the stage of sleep from which he is called to wakefulness. The difficulty in arousing people from sleep during the early part of the night may reflect the fact that the deep slow-wave stage 4 occurs most frequently in that initial period. Since people may be able to learn to discriminate between REM sleep and stage 2, perhaps the discrimination can be further refined. A person might then learn to awaken from a stage of light sleep, an optimum point on the cycle, for it seems very likely that awakening comes more easily from some phases of sleep than others.

Summary

Voluntary control over sleep behavior and, indeed, some facets of waking consciousness, have come into systematic investigation only recently. Only a bare beginning has been made in the study of sleep behavior itself. Even in this partial review, it must be clear that there are many difficulties inherent in this area of study. Not least among them may be our difficulty in defining sleep. Some people can respond to the outside world without showing apparent EEG changes in their sleep, yet others show rhythms resembling those we identify with waking. Moreover, people have been known to sleepwalk out of the EEGs of deep sleep, or to show sleeping brain waves while seemingly wide awake. The behavior of lying still with eyes closed is not enough to tell us that a person is asleep, and sleeplike brain waves may be contradicted by apparently alert behavior. The fact that there appear to be two extremely different kinds of sleep and that behavior during REM sleep often differs from the rest, does not help to settle the problem. We have, however, begun to recognize these problems, and that is the sign of a giant stride into a region of human life, of activity and consciousness, that never before seemed so rich.

Although the conditioning of brain wave sequences and the exploration of introspective development may seem Olympian and distant from practical application, such studies may ultimately offer powerful new techniques to the medical doctor and to the psychotherapist and psychiatrist through instruction in physical and mental control. We have discovered that people can discriminate between one phase of sleep and another, can accept some information during sleep, and can communicate with the outside world. They can learn to control states of consciousness that they couldn't previously identify and for which they had no awareness. The EEG, used as a feedback system, may make it possible to instruct people in the verbally incommunicable. Most of these findings cannot be applied at once, but progress has been rapid, for the work cited here has been accomplished largely in the last 5 years. It is clear that the feats of a Hamid Bey hold some considerable interest for us still, although in a new light. Self-sovereignty and full access to one's own richness of consciousness is the supposed epitome of the cultivated man, yet the discipline of body and mind that might mould such an ideal have long been neglected by the Judeo-Christian majority of the Western World.

Chapter VII.
The Dream State of REM

Once upon a time, before 1952, most people thought that dreams were rare events, perhaps caused by bodily discomfort or aching conscience, by trauma, sensory stimulation, or the insurgence of an unruly subconscious. The discovery that all people dream every night came as a surprise to many although a large number of classical studies had already heralded the finding. Like many developments in science, a long progression of researchers composed the prelude to the work of this decade although the earlier work attracted less public attention.

The germinal studies, from which much of modern sleep research has burgeoned, began innocuously enough at the University of Chicago where Dr. Nathaniel Kleitman devoted himself single-mindedly to the study of sleep. Dr. Eugene Aserinsky, then a graduate student working with Kleitman, turned attention toward phenomena that had been spotted before and never thoroughly studied. Aserinsky, studying the movements of sleeping infants, was arrested by the fact that the slow rolling movements of the eyes would stop

193

periodically, for intervals. He began to watch adults and saw that there were recurrent intervals of body quiescence when the eyes began making rapid jerky movements beneath the closed lids. At that time it was a curious and startling observation, and it took some doing on the part of a graduate student to demonstrate that this periodic activity did indeed occur in sleep. When Aserinsky and Kleitman watched sleeping volunteers they saw that the rapid eye movements (REMs) occurred periodically, at a time when there were sharp increases in respiration and heart rate and the EEG showed a low-voltage, desynchronized pattern very different from the rolling waves of deep sleep (Aserinsky and Kleitman, 1953, 1955; Kleitman, 1960, 1963).

Back in the 1930's, shrewd observers indicated that this EEG pattern meant dreaming qualitatively different from dreaming in other stages of sleep but the time was not then ripe for a surge of corroborating research on this phase of sleep. When Aserinsky and Kleitman awakened volunteers during this REM and EEG pattern, subjects almost always narrated a dream, while awakenings at other periods of sleep rarely evoked such reports. Dr. William C. Dement, then also a graduate student at Chicago, pursued the finding, affirming the coincidence of dreaming with the REM and low-voltage EEG pattern (Dement and Kleitman 1957). Subsequently he noted the same pattern in the sleep of cats, a finding confirmed by Dr. Michel Jouvet of the Faculty of Medicine in Lyon (Jouvet, 1960). At this point two major paths of dream exploration had begun in the animal laboratory of neurophysiology and in the EEG laboratory where human volunteers came to sleep out the night.

Nobody could have predicted how rapidly sleep research would capture the scientific imagination. Where a few men with solitary persistence had concentrated on the overlooked third of life, in 10 years there followed a new generation of scientists, many of whom elected sleep as their province of research. From the start the arresting differences between the REM intervals and the rest of sleep suggested that REM was a unique physiological and psychological state. The physiology, itself, began to show a unique configuration first emerging from the studies of Dr. Frederick Snyder and his associates at NIH (Snyder, 1960).

Since 1952 so much data has come pouring out of the laboratories that it cannot be recounted in a small space. A sampling may indicate what we have learned about the amount of REM dreaming in humans and animals and what it may indicate about the evolution of the mammal brain, the development of the normal infant brain, mental hygiene, and mental illness. Many of our clues about the physiology of dreaming have come in bits and pieces, as have our data showing the nature of brain activity during dreaming, with implications that may aid our understanding of mental illness. Although the bits and pieces do not fit together as a neat whole, they have been generally congruent, linking activity of body, mind, and behavior in a way that has advanced the study of human behavior another step out of the dark ages of phenomenology. There is no neat way to isolate research in neurophysiology from research on bodily changes during dreaming, or personality factors, nor to isolate the chemistry of dreaming, or behavioral data, and so the grouping used to describe studies of the dreaming state is somewhat arbitrary.

The REM Cycle

Back in the olden days of dream research, little more than a decade ago, two very remarkable facts were discovered. Today they are taken for granted, but at that time masses of data and many confirmations were required to persuade the scientists that they really had found what they thought they had found. Everybody dreamt every night, and moreover, they dreamt in regular cycles, each for roughly the same amount of time (Dement, 1965). Subjectively it is easier to think of dreaming as infrequent, because, in part, memory for dreams is so brief. Yet the assortment of students and housewives who were paid to sleep in Abbot Hall at the University of Chicago gave richly detailed dream narratives when awakened during REM periods. As Dement and other investigators repeatedly awakened volunteers it became clear that young adults had a similar pattern of vivid dream episodes. About 90 minutes after falling asleep they would rise into a REM state, usually for a short period, about 10 minutes, then sink down into deep sleep for about an hour before rising again for a longer dream period. Hundreds and hundreds of people have now been recorded, and the average young adult seems to dream about 20–25 percent of his sleeping time, in five or so REM periods, at roughly hourly intervals. Individuals appear to have somewhat distinctive patterns, and some investigators can look at a person's EEG record of several nights' sleep and predict when he will start dreaming, and for how long.

The very discovery of an outside handle to a person's dreams set a blaze in the imaginations of psychologists and psychiatrists. Was this EEG state akin to the hallucinating states of psychotics or the DT's of alcoholics? Were certain psychotic symptoms merely displaced dreaming? If everybody dreamed a certain amount each night, what happened when a person couldn't dream?

REM Deprivation

During the mid-1950's, Dr. Dement, working with Dr. Charles Fisher at Mount Sinai Hospital in New York, began the first of a series of dream deprivation experiments. Volunteers, carefully observed and questioned, and under strict rules not to take alcohol or drugs or naps, were allowed to sleep their usual sleep in the laboratory—except for REM periods. At the first sign of rapid eye movement and EEG desynchronized pattern, the subject was awakened, then permitted to go back to sleep. For five successive nights the volunteers were awakened in this manner. Although they had gotten about 6 hours of sleep, some of them complained of psychological discomfort, began to eat more than usual, and suffered anxiety. One subject quit the study after several days in an apparent panic. This did not happen to the control subjects whose equivalent awakenings took place in non-REM periods (Dement, 1960). The initial study, which has since been reexecuted in many variations, created a great flare of excitement. It suggested that people needed to dream. Not only did deprived subjects complain of some psychological discomfort, but on each successive night they attempted to dream more often. After their stint of dream deprivation, when they slept undisturbed in the laboratory, they dreamed about 60 percent more than they had on baseline nights. They appeared to be making up for lost dreams.

Initially, the psychological facet of the need to dream captured the most attention. Deprive a person of his dreams, the study suggested, and he begins to suffer psychological abnormalities. This interpretation coincided nicely with Freud's theory that dreaming formed the safety valve of mankind, permitting an expression for the many drives and impulses that civilized man must repress. Many subsequent dream-deprivation studies have thrown this interpretation into question. Dement, himself, and many others have sometimes failed to notice any marked psychological changes even after more thorough and extended deprivation. But the need to dream—as expressed in ever increasing attempts to dream and in a huge and unambiguous orgy of compensatory REM time following deprivation—has been seen in every deprivation experiment, human or animal. Dr. Charles Sawyer and his associates at UCLA deprived rabbits of REM sleep by leaving them in a chamber where a hissing noise was continuously played. When the noise was turned off, the rabbits appeared to make up lost REM time with more frequent and longer REM periods. Dr. Michel Jouvet and his associates in Lyon have deprived cats of REM sleep for as long as 26 days. Subsequently allowed uninterrupted sleep, the cats spent about 60 percent of their time in the REM state and fell directly into that state from waking. This compensatory dreaming has been observed in people, among them dexedrine addicts and alcoholics who have been withdrawn from dream-suppressing drugs. It has been seen among the totally sleep deprived and among some psychotics after periods of reduced REM time. The need to dream appears to be uniform, or perhaps one should say, the need for REM sleep.

Today, with mounting evidence from animal studies, it appears that the need for REM sleep must be more than a psychological need. The dreaming of the REM state is a physiological as well as a psychological process. Indeed, it has been thought that the psychological disruptions observed in some volunteers after dream deprivation are actually the signals of a physical penalty that may have to be paid if the REM cycle is prevented for too long a time. Nevertheless, it is interesting that people have varied in their reactions in the several deprivation studies so far. The very fact that some people show effects and others do not raises questions that are germane to a wide variety of human studies in psychology, and may be worth examining as an instance of the uncertainties facing scientists within the broader context.

Why have some subjects felt anxious, empty, hungry, unable to concentrate, a few of them even extremely unsettled after a degree of REM loss that had no such effects upon subjects in other studies? Possibly, in some of the initial and short studies the experimenters did not see in their screening of volunteers that they were in a state of fatigue. Subjects may have been more anxious to begin with than was apparent on testing. There is another possibility, albeit unlikely. Sometimes even the most cautious experimenter may inadvertently reveal his expectations by cues so subtle that the subjects will live up to an expected role without even knowing they are doing so. This has been a pitfall in many studies of hypnosis, but it seems an unlikely explanation here, because animals deprived of REM sleep have shown pronounced behavioral symptoms.

Cats, deprived of their activated REM phase for long enough, show very bizarre behavior disorders. Cats have been deprived of REM sleep in several ways. They have been placed upon a stone or other object surrounded by water. This permitted them slow-wave sleep, but they would topple into cold water whenever their neck and head muscles relaxed at the onset of REM sleep. In some studies they have been awakened by an attendant and set upon their feet the moment their EEGs and muscle tonus signaled the onset of REM periods. Jouvet has observed distinctions between deprived and normal laboratory cats, even after moderate deprivation. The deprived animals were, in Jouvet's expression, tired, sad cats. Visitors to the Lyon laboratory were able to pick out cats who had been REM deprived a year earlier because they were so subdued and unaggressive. More recently, Dement and Jouvet have subjected cats to prolonged deprivation periods of 30–

70 days. These cats have exhibited a variety of disturbances. Some have become "hungry," eating abnormally, restless and indiscriminately hypersexual. They have acted as if their basic drives were enhanced by the deprivation.

In studying human beings, the experimenters have always terminated the deprivation long before there were such abnormal signs out of apprehension that REM loss might cause irreversible damage. Dement and his associates have been studying cats under partial deprivation and severe deprivation to see whether there is damage to the nervous system. When a cat's nervous system is in any way "poisoned" there will be a discernible difference in its EEG after hearing a click. One of the tests for REM loss damage has been a series of recordings from the cochlear nucleus of cats. This is a first relay station for the sound impulse traveling upward in the brain. A first study has shown that the EEG response changes considerably in the REM deprived cats, returning to normal after the animal has been allowed REM sleep. Control animals, awakened on the same schedule as the deprived cats, showed no change in EEG response (Dewson et al., 1965). Other signs of altered sensitivity within regions of the brain may accompany REM loss, perhaps associated with biochemical changes. These may indeed be related to the behavioral changes noted.

Notwithstanding the animal studies, there have been several dream deprivation studies conducted with human volunteers, which have shown apparently conflicting results. Subjected to 5 days of REM deprivation, and not total deprivation at that, volunteers reported irritability, emptiness, anxiety and other symptoms (Dement, 1960). Yet a person in a later study conducted by the same experimenters, endured 13 consecutive nights of dream deprivation with few signs of changes.

More recently, Dement and his associates went through a grueling vigil in order to deprive three subjects of all REM sleep for 16 days. This time the subjects were awakened the moment muscle tone disappeared under the chin, an event that usually precedes the other signals of a REM period. After eight nights the first subject was trying to dream so often and it was so hard to wrestle him awake that it became impossible to deprive him of REM sleep without totally depriving him of sleep. He would start dreaming the moment he was allowed to close his eyes and fall asleep. The next volunteer was given dexedrine to suppress dreaming. He, too, began dreaming more and more often. Soon the investigators had to awaken him incessantly. By the 15th night he was dreaming as soon as he closed his eyes, a behavior seen among narcoleptics, certain psychotics, or after drug withdrawal. By this time he had changed from a taciturn, compunctious, moral person into a blue-streak talker, an unreliable subject, a man who wanted to sit in a nightclub without ordering drinks until he was thrown out. On his first night of recovery he dreamed 120 percent more than usual and reverted back to his normal self. The third subject showed a personality transformation after 14 nights of deprivation, and the experiment was terminated after 16 nights. On the next night he dreamed 160 percent more

202

than his usual REM quota, and he, too reverted to his usual self (Dement, 1965).

Another subject deprived of dreams for 16 nights by Dement and Fisher had shown no psychotic symptoms, but he evinced obviously disturbed behavior, memory disturbances, time sense distortions, preoccupations, and an inability to work. He sat around in a stupor most of the day, yet when he was being tested or interviewed, he managed to mobilize his forces. This is probably an important issue in many psychological studies, for as everyone knows from experience, it is possible to be exhausted, distraught, and largely immobilized, yet summon up all one's resources at a critical moment and give a good performance.

All in all there have been few studies of prolonged dream deprivation. This is understandable because it is a monumental strain on the endurance of investigators. Each subject must be monitored continuously, day and night. The experimenter must keep a tense vigil throughout several nights of baseline recording, then maintain a split-second alertness throughout the consecutive deprivation nights, followed by the nights of recovery sleep.

One recent deprivation study of two young men was prompted by the discrepancies in psychological reactions (Kales et al., 1964). The subjects were under constant observation, and were deprived of REM periods in two separate experiments. For 6 nights, the rapid eye movements formed the awakening signals, whereas for 10 consecutive nights the loss of muscle tonus was used as the alarm clock. In both studies neither psychological testing nor direct observation revealed any significant changes. Both volunteers reported vivid dreams and fragments when awakened, suggesting that they obtained several seconds of dreaming even before loss of muscle tone signaled the investigators to awaken them. The investigators conjectured that this brief period contained a great deal of compressed and perhaps accelerated dreaming, and they concluded that despite marked REM deprivation they were not really dream depriving subjects.

There is still another possibility. Individuals may vary considerably in the amount of REM loss they can stand before they begin to show palpable signs. Although researchers have been careful to avoid accepting volunteers who are neurotic, overtired, or in an obviously precarious mental state, there is a great range of constitutional and personality differences in humankind. Members of the U.S. astronaut team, who have demonstrated a certain hale and rugged capacity to withstand all manner of stresses differ from other members of the population who are nevertheless quite healthy. People differ considerably in their response to a simple test such as placing a hand in cold water for a brief time. Perhaps the different responses to intervals of REM deprivation reflect another dimension on which human beings vary, and the point of psychological susceptibility may vary both among people and within the same person during different stages of his life. One might still expect that there would be a limit beyond which an individual could not suffer REM loss without palpable signs.

If there is an element of individual differences in tolerance to dream loss, and indeed a wide distribution of mental-constitutional traits, one might expect to see a similar diversity in animals, some evidence in animal studies of marked diversity within the same species. There have been a number of cases bearing on this point, and one which is particularly relevant.

Personality and EEG Differences in Cats

Although we tend to treat animals the same in the laboratory, everyone is aware that cats differ from one another much as people do. A demonstration of these differences has been part of a long research program conducted by Dr. Barbara Brown and her associates at the Sepulveda V. A. Hospital. The behavioral traits of 100 cats were categorized by a Q-sort technique, and subsequent studies showed that distinctive EEG characteristics occurred with each of the major "personality" groups. The purpose of this classification was to obtain some baseline of an animal's behavior before testing on him psychotropic drugs in doses comparable to those that would be given the human patient. Two striking studies will illustrate the extent of the EEG-behavioral differences observed among these cats. Usually, when an animal explores a new cage, orienting himself so to speak, he will show a theta rhythm from the hippocampus. The frequency of theta decreases as the cats become adapted to the new cage. Cats who had been categorized as "average," when placed in a strange recording cage spent the least time exploring before settling down to sleep, and showed their theta rhythm at this time, but it soon vanished as they adapted. Cats who were categorized as "anxious, or withdrawn" spent considerable time exploring the new cage, and showed a great deal of theta, at a very high frequency usually seen in activated (REM) sleep. Cats described as "overly outgoing" also spent a long time exploring and adapting, showed a great deal of theta, but of a lower frequency than the rhythm of the other cats.

Usually, during activated or dreaming sleep the cat again shows the hippocampal theta rhythm. Cats scored as "average" showed theta sleep the first time they were in the recording cage. Both "outgoing" and "withdrawn or anxious" animals took as long as four or six sessions in the recording cage before they showed theta during sleep. Minimal theta during orienting, and the appearance of theta during sleep might indeed be said to be a sign of quick adaptation, theta perhaps representing a fundamental behavioral signpost.

Differences between the "average" cats, and the "outgoing" or "withdrawn" animals reasserted themselves when the animals were given a small amount of alcohol. Within the first 20–30 minutes after their drink, all of the "outgoing" were drowsing or asleep, although some of the animals showed and awake EEG. Similarly, all of the "withdrawn" cats were asleep within a half hour after taking their drink, but these cats showed a slow and sleeplike EEG in the experimental situation, even before sleep. By contrast, the "average" cats were awake and alert for 2 hours after their drink, and although none slept, some showed a sleep EEG while others showed an EEG of waking. Behaviorally, in any event, the "average" cats reacted to alcohol very differently from the deviant animals.

Experiments with REM deprived cats suggest that there may be some difference among the animals, but this has not been the focus of these studies. These studies are yielding essential information that cannot be obtained from human studies. One such study may be important in understanding what happens when a person continuously suffers a small reduction in REM dreaming, either because he has a sleep disturbance or mental illness, or because he takes drugs or is alcoholic.

Partial Dream Deprivation

One research study on human volunteers has suggested that there may be differences in the way people compensate for partial dream loss, certainly over short intervals (Sampson, 1965).

Dr. Harold Sampson of Mount Zion Hospital, San Francisco, has been watching for any detectable psychological changes that might come from partial dream deprivation, but a deprivation not occasioned by constant awakenings or by drugs. Subjects in this study go for several consecutive nights with only 2½ hours of sleep. Here individuals differ greatly in the rapidity with which they begin to dream and how much of their sleep is taken up in dreaming. For instance, one person dreamed for a full hour on his second night of reduced sleep, but only 10 minutes the next night, and showed almost no compensatory dreaming on recovery nights of full sleep. Another person managed to dream for only 1 minute on the first deprivation night, for 15 minutes on the next, and about 40 minutes on the third night. These signs may be reflecting constitutional differences in reacting to dream loss.

Another, perhaps related, incident of individual variation was observed in an experiment that was, roughly speaking, designed to see whether a person compensates for 5 nights of total REM deprivation and for 20 nights of 25 percent REM deprivation with the same amount of recovery REM time. After 20 nights of partial (25 percent) REM loss, 1 subject showed an increase that would have been compatible with 5 days of total deprivation. However, something very interesting had been noticed during the 10 consecutive nights during which the experimenters were computing the subject's normal quota of REM sleep.

Two subjects showed a slight increase in the percentage of REM sleep throughout these 10 baseline nights, while 2 other subjects gave every evidence of a constant REM quota after their first 2 nights in the laboratory. This suggests that it may be necessary to observe some laboratory volunteers for a very long time before concluding what percentage of their sleep time is spent in the REM period (Dement et al., 1965). Whether these differences reflect reactions to the laboratory situation, to events in the person's life, or to changes in schedule, diet, or physiology, they illustrate some of the difficulties inherent in dream-sleep research.

For all the individual diversity in reaction to dream loss, and for all the variance seen in animals, one factor remains unchanged. An individual spends a fairly constant portion of his sleep in REM dreaming. When his REM quota is reduced, whether it occurs as a result of fever, of anxiety, of alcohol, drugs, or awakening, he will dream more on subsequent nights.

Of course, when an experimenter deprives an individual of REM sleep, or when a person deprives himself either through illness, by cutting down on sleep, or by drugs—he is not just losing dreams. The brilliant episodes of inward experience are summoned by the activity of the brain, and are accompanied by bodily processes. The lost intervals are not only psychological, as rapid eye movements, themselves, might have suggested. The process in which our most memorable dreaming seems to occur is an integrated neural process, related to the surging of our emotions, the behavior of our bodies. Within the experience of the dream itself, the memories we summon, the euphoria or rage we feel must follow some laws by which the central nervous system and indeed our entire body and being operate (Fair, 1963).

Muscle Tone

When the REM period is excerpted from even a single night of sleep, a huge variety of body activities must go with it, for the unique properties of the REM dream period are not restricted to the brain. The brain's peculiar activity at this time is correlated with effects throughout the muscles and in the autonomic system.

The most dramatic demonstration of changes in muscle tone is the cataplectic fit of a narcoleptic who goes through no slow transitions but falls directly into a REM state and collapses like jelly. The relaxation of sleep involves a decrease of elec-

209

trical activity in muscles throughout the body. These changes have been observed by many but were recently mapped in a thorough way by a team of UCLA researchers (Jacobson et al., 1964; Dement, 1965). They found that the body muscles do not show marked changes from one stage of sleep to another. Clearly, they retain some potential, because people do move and turn. During stage 4 some people even get up and walk in their sleep. Many people have noticed that a person turns and moves as he approaches a dream period, like a person settling in a theater seat before the curtain. Then he is relatively quiet. By using surface electrodes on volunteers, the UCLA team watched the changing activity levels of 29 muscles during sleep. Occasionally there would be bursts, some of these corresponding with twitches during REM periods, but in general then the activity levels were low. At the onset of REM sleep, however, the head and neck muscles show a sharp decrease in tonus. This is such a reliable phenomenon that the muscle under the chin has been used as a REM alarm clock.

By placing an electrode on the chin muscle, its sudden decrease in electrical activity can be used to activate a switch, telling an experimenter in another room when an animal or person has started dreaming. The same technique has been useful with small babies, permitting a count of their REM time without burdening them with other electrodes.

Because certain head muscles lose tonus at the onset of REM sleep, it is perfectly apparent whenever a rabbit starts to dream. This is the one time when its ears flop. Ordinarily the creature will stretch out in a number of positions to sleep, ears held straight back, but during the REM state they suddenly droop.

The picture of an animal in this phase of sleep is familiar to any pet owner. The paws, tail, and whiskers occasionally twitch, the animal may lick or suck or even emit barks or cries. Sometimes his extremities are slightly convulsed in myoclonic jerks. Occasionally penile erections occur. The ears may twitch and the nictitating membranes almost completely cover the pupils of the eyes. Breathing may be irregular, and the eyeballs seem to move in short rapid jerks. This is the picture observed in dogs, cats, rats, rabbits, monkeys, and man. Dr. Frederick Snyder of NIMH has recently observed that the opossum, a most primitive animal, shows REM sleep. Signs of REM sleep have been found in all mammals investigated: in the lamb, ass, goat, even in birds.

Physiological Excitation

During these periods of REM sleep animals and men seem to be swept by waves of physiological activity, storms of neural excitement. The ripples of activity on the surface are more noticeable than eye movements, and could be seen by any careful observer. They did not attract attention and study in the past, partly because people were not looking, and partly no doubt because bedclothes obscured body movement. Active sleep is quite apparent in infants. Out of a quiescent serenity an infant can be seen, suddenly frowning, sucking, grimacing, his breathing uneven, his fists waving and uncurling, feet kicking. Anybody can see these signs. Although periods of "disturbed" sleep, probably REM periods, had been observed in the 1920's by a clinician who speculated that they were associated with dreams and instances of cardiac catastrophe, no careful sleep studies of heart rate and respiration were made at that time. There was no correlation between the EEG and "disturbed sleep" (MacWilliams). The intuition was nevertheless a sound one, for it is during the early morning hours, the time when people have their longest dream periods, that inexplicable heart attacks sometimes occur. During early studies of the REM period in adults, Aserinsky and Kleitman observed that the heart rate and respiration rate seemed to increase in these intervals. The physiology of the dream state warranted a much closer examination, and it was Dr. Frederick Snyder and his associates at NIMH, who initiated the now extensive exploration, starting in the late 1950's. As their research program has begun to indicate, the physiology of the REM state has many ramifications for medicine, for the treatment of cardiac patients, epileptics, and many patients whose symptoms appear to be exacerbated during those particular hours in which REM sleep prevails.

Cardiorespiratory Changes

A closer look at the heart rate, the blood pressure, and the respiration of sleeping adults revealed no simple and striking increases during REM sleep, for the increased levels were relatively small. The overall nightly pattern, observed in a study of 12 young men and women, in-

212

dicated that systolic blood pressure begins to drop at the onset of sleep reaching a minimum in about 2 hours, and rising progressively back to its original level during the rest of the night. Respiration and heart rate dropped continuously as the night wore on (Snyder 1960, 1962, 1964).

If these cardiorespiratory functions did not show large and uniform increases during REM sleep, they showed another pattern that is perhaps more alarming to the clinician apprehensive about nighttime cardiac crises. During REM periods the systolic blood pressure, pulse, and respiration fluctuated, sometimes wildly, an erratic pattern that sometimes sent blood pressure above any levels observed during the quiet waking intervals before sleep. (Snyder et al., 1964). Nightlong measurements of pulse rate and blood pressure had been taken by recording pulse sounds from a microphone taped on the ankle, and an automatically inflated leg cuff, a laborious collection task that was followed by an even more laborious data analysis (Snyder et al., 1963). The REM periods were, indeed, intervals of marked variability, a finding that has since been confirmed by other investigators (Kamiya, 1961; Shapiro et al., 1964).

Whether this variability is related to the emotions of dreaming, is triggered by excitations from the central nervous system, or by a combination of mechanisms—it is a finding of considerable interest. Systolic blood pressure, as measured by an arm or leg cuff, is the pressure of blood expelled from the heart by its contraction. This pressure is reflected in the expansion of arteries and veins. In the healthy person with a normal heart, the systolic surge is followed by decreased pressure in direct proportion. This is the diastolic phase of pressure that occurs when the heart expands and the chambers fill with blood. The intervals of contraction and expansion are reflected in the pulsing of the blood, from which we detect the rate at which the heart is pumping. The relation between pulse rate, blood pressure, and rate of respiration is complicated and not well understood. Variations of heart rate and blood pressure often occurred during fluctuations in breathing but sometimes they were independent (Snyder et al., 1964). These occasionally dramatic and sudden excursions in the heart rate and blood pressure may offer a clue to the nighttime heart attack and cardiac failure during sleep. Many people have supposed that violent dreams might be the cause of such attacks, and a number of investigators have observed that particularly intense dreams may be accompanied by more eye movements, and greater changes in respiration. It is early to say whether the emotionality and violence of dreams are always matched by greater changes in these outward bodily indicators (Snyder, 1960, 1965).

The radical physiological fluctuations that were observed by Snyder and others present more of a problem than would progressive increases in blood pressure, etc. In hypertensive patients, for instance, it is true that high blood pressure is worrisome, but the more dangerous tendency is often that of sudden and enormous shifts in blood pressure which are hard to prevent and control, even by sympathectomy or drugs.

It is clear, given the clinical ramifications, why

investigators have wanted to obtain very precise measurements of blood pressure during sleep. Direct measures of arterial blood pressure and blood flow might be obtained continuously throughout the night by using implanted catheters. This is a difficult and touchy procedure, but it has been accomplished in the monkey, revealing the pattern observed in man—great variability during REM sleep (Stoyva et al., 1965). Similarly, heart rate and respiration varied during REM sleep.

Oxygen Consumption

Some recent findings by Dr. Eugene Aserinsky may help to explain this picture. At the onset of each REM period respiration is regular, but it becomes shallow breathing. When breathing becomes very shallow, there is less oxygen in the blood. At times, during REM periods, arterial oxygen saturation drops below the point that a person would tolerate were he awake and holding his breath. This may trigger an acceleration, an increase in the respiratory rate. It is not clear exactly what causes this incredibly shallow breathing. However, there may be some connection between the depth of respiration and the heart rate, in which shallow breathing is accompanied by a transient slowing of the heart.

The observation of peculiar respiration patterns during sleep, relatively even and regular during slow-wave phases, variable during REM periods, led to many questions about the mechanisms that might be causing them. The consumption of oxygen is an important part of the body's energy metabolism, and one method of looking indirectly at metabolism has been to examine the exchange of inhaled and exhaled gases. This is the basis of the rough and ready basal metabolism test which measures oxygen consumption. Dr. Aserinsky has used an oximeter, attached to the ear lobe of a well trained sleeping volunteer, and a face mask that filtered out exhaled carbon dioxide and oxygen. By this method he found that the oxygen level decreased sharply and reached its lowest levels during REM sleep, a sharp decrease not observed during slow-wave sleep. This may seem related to the shallow breathing, subsequently found during REM sleep. On the other hand, there was no evidence of pronounced changes in carbon dioxide in the periods leading up to the REM periods. A recent study of gas exchange, in another laboratory, suggests that there may be some accumulation of carbon dioxide in the body during the intervals between REM periods. These apparent inconsistencies reflect the use of different instruments, and different handling of the data, understandable in an area demanding such difficult techniques.

One recent search for the clues to metabolism during sleep by examining gas exchange has employed a temperature and humidity controlled metabolic chamber. Thirty subjects have been studied within this chamber, as they slept through the night, under a plastic hood. Air was continuously pumped into the hood, and analyzed for oxygen consumption and carbon dioxide excretion. An initial analysis suggests that there is a relationship between metabolism and the stages of sleep observed on the EEG. Oxygen utilization appeared to be greatest during REM sleep and least during stage 4, and carbon dioxide appeared to be accumulating during the intervals between REM periods (Brebbia and Altshuler, 1965).

Beginning with the outward signs of eye movements, respiration, muscle tonus, etc., scientists saw the clues that the dream state, REM sleep, had certain physiological properties that were different from the rest of sleep. Why do respiration and blood pressure show certain peculiar changes? Why does the gas exchange seem to change? The questions have led inward.

Brain Temperature

Two laboratories, working independently, have seen evidence that there are portions of the brain which rise in temperature during REM sleep. Sleeping rabbits, implanted with small thermocouples in the preoptic region of the hypothalamus, have shown a waxing and waning of brain temperature, considerable variation during sleep. During slow-wave sleep, the brain temperature dropped, but it rose sharply during episodes of REM or activated sleep, sometimes reaching temperatures higher than those of waking arousal. Implants in other brain regions also showed similar temperature fluctuations, but more slowly, whereas measurements taken in the skin of the neck and body did not show temperature changes parallel to those of the brain. This suggested that the forebrain, and particularly the hypothalamus, might be areas in which there is a great deal of metabolic activity during REM sleep (Kawamura and Sawyer, 1965).

A similar conclusion was drawn from a study

of cats. Cats with thermistors implanted in the cortex or hypothalamus indicated the onset of REM periods with a considerable rise in brain temperature. Moreover, the rising brain temperature was correlated with diminishing amplitude of the brain waves, suggesting that the dimension of the brain waves, themselves, might give some index of brain metabolism (Rechtschaffen et al., 1965). Once again, judging from notable increases in brain temperature and their implications for brain metabolism, it seems that the REM state is curiously different from the rest of sleep, bearing many resemblances to waking.

Biochemical Changes

Metabolism is, of course, a very general term and perhaps misleading on that account, for body and brain metabolism encompass the multitude of systems that break down food, air, and other substances into the useful components to provide energy, or construct other chemicals, repair cells, etc. A host of biochemical transformations are constantly occurring and interacting throughout the body, throughout life. Reasonably, investigators have suspected that the peculiar REM period must be accompanied by diverse biochemical changes. Small changes, especially in human subjects, are hard to detect, and offer a technical challenge that often outstrips our present laboratory capabilities. However, a start has been made in the search for some of the more relevant and perhaps related chemical changes, and this new body of work has been reviewed by Dr. Arnold Mandell of UCLA (Mandell, 1965).

A number of subjects have learned to sleep with a catheter in their arm, and it has been possible to scan the rise and fall of free fatty acids in the blood during sleep. These substances reach peak concentration around the middle of the night and drop to a nadir before waking. Their variation over the course of the night may turn out to be correlated with the occurrences of REM periods (Scott, 1964).

Nightlong blood samplings have been obtained from other catheter-wearing subjects, in order to trace the course of certain stress hormones, the 17-hydroxycorticosteroids. These steroids show a pronounced effect upon the central nervous system, and when they are not in adequate production can induce an inability to concentrate, and restlessness. They appear to be most concentrated in the blood during the early morning hours, before awakening, and in lowest concentration at night, showing a correspondence with the circadian rhythm. The interesting pattern observed in a study of six subjects was that the rise in 17–OHCS was not gradual, but that it occurred in a series of jumps during the latter part of the night's sleep. These elevations came in intervals of 1–2 hours, and there was some correlation with REM periods. One pattern was clear for all subjects: The hormone level during the second half of the night was four times the level in the first half—a ratio in striking correspondence with the percentage of sleep devoted to REM, which was five times as great during the second half of the night. Although these hormone levels may not turn out to play a role in causing REM sleep, they may suggest one link in a biochemical chain, part of a hypothetical and biological clock that triggers the activity we know as the REM dream state (Weitzman et al., 1965).

Various hormonal fluctuations may be associated with a number of curious bodily changes during REM sleep. Some hormones, for example, play an important role within the gastric system. Here is another area that has shown some interesting activity during sleep. Patients with duodenal ulcers, for example, have been known to exhibit high gastric secretion at night. Very recently a group of investigators looked into the patterns of patients with duodenal ulcers, with the hunch that their high nighttime gastric secretions might be related with REM dreaming. Patients and normal controls all slept with tubes from which stomach contents were sampled, while polygraph recordings were taken. The ulcer patients showed a significant increase in gastric secretion during REM periods, whereas the controls had a low secretion rate throughout the night, and one that did not differ greatly whether they were awake, in dreaming, or nondreaming sleep (Armstrong et al., 1965).

The recent and growing evidence of pronounced biochemical changes, coinciding with the REM period, may not be knit together for some time to come, but it has struck off a surge of investigation that already shows some clinical interest.

Erection Cycles

As people look more closely at the physical dreamer, it is evident that the bizarre images, the travelogues of the mind, are not the only strange events of the REM period, but that the entire person must be swept by unusual excitations. One of the more obvious of these signs is the penile erection that slightly precedes almost every REM period in males, from infancy into great age. The phenomenon of nightly erections was described by three German researchers two decades ago as occurring at intervals of roughly 85 minutes and lasting some 25 minutes. This sounded so much like the distribution of REM periods that Ian Oswald of Cambridge University began to study the phenomenon. His measuring instruments precluded a reliable correlation; however, a correlation between REM periods and erections has been made recently by Dr. Charles Fisher, Joseph Gross, and Joseph Zuch at Mount Sinai Hospital in New York. An initial study of 17 subjects indicated that erections preceded rapid eye movements and lasted throughout 95 percent of the REM periods. Recent studies have indicated that this phenomenon is not altered by recency of sexual orgasm, and it does not seem to stem from overtly sexual dream content. If 95 percent of the REM periods are accompanied by erection, then the odd dream periods need explanation. Instances of sudden detumescence appear to be related to dreams of severe anxiety, and total absence of erection may be related to fatigue and anxiety (Fisher et al., 1965, Karacan et al., 1965). It has been observed among animals and man that intense emotional excitement, not specifically sexual, can be accompanied by erection. Perhaps this is a discharge overflow from intense

221

neural excitement occurring within drive-related centers that are activated in the dreaming brain.

The Eye Movements

One of the most puzzling of the dream accompaniments is the physical signpost by which it was detected, the rapid eye movements themselves. Why do the eyes move as if they are watching events on a screen or reading? The obvious answer seemed at first to be that the eyes were scanning the dream images. A number of investigators have reported that there seemed to be more actual eye movements accompanying dreams of events that in real life would require frequent shifts of gaze (Berger and Oswald, 1962). Several investigators sought to find out whether the eyes moved when a person merely imagined some activity. Dr. G. H. Deckert showed a swinging pendulum to subjects, then asked them to close their eyes and imagine it. Their eye movements, when they were imagining the movement, closely resembled the actual watching of the pendulum (Deckert, 1964). A further study by Dr. Barbara B. Brown and her associates suggested that the eye movements during such a recall would slightly exaggerate or diminish the original, real motion, and that these movements occurred both in people who deliberately experience visual imagery and those who cannot (Brown et al., 1964). Similar evidences have come from others (Antrobus et al., 1964).

If the overt eye movements of dreaming indicated the scanning of images on an interior screen, they might not be expected of the blind, especially the congenitally blind. Drs. R. Berger, P. Olley, and I. Oswald found no rapid eye movements or reports of visual imagery in the dreams of congenitally blind people, although they did exist in people who had been blind from 3–15 years (Berger et al., 1962). Drs. William Offenkrantz and Edward Wolpert did see one instance of rapid eye movements in a congenitally blind person whose dreams were not visual, and recent studies of people with lifelong blindness have indicated that they do have rapid eye movements during stage one "dreaming" sleep. It would seem that previous failures to record REMs in the congenitally blind have been due to deficiencies in the recording method. (Gross et al., 1965).

In 1960, Drs. Howard Roffwarg, W. C. Dement, Joseph Muzio, and Charles Fisher carefully awakened volunteers after particular eye movements, and asked for detailed accounts of the dream event. Another investigator, who did not see the record of eye movements, was given the dream story and told to map out and space the eye movements that would match it. These tracings matched the actual eye movement record with great accuracy. This work and further studies correlating eye motion with dream event suggested that the eyes were indeed following dream events (Roffwarg et al., 1962).

Although the eye movements may be related to the moving pictures of the mind, the response may not resemble the voluntary action of watching a real tennis game nor even with eyes closed, imagining a game. A number of very different findings bear on this point. First of all, some of the eye movements recorded during dreaming are so large and furious they would be inconceivable as voluntary movements in waking life. (Oswald, 1962). Rapid conjugate eye movements can be caused by artificially changing the electrophysiological state of the frontal cortex (Rassmussen and Penfield). Animal studies, primarily studies of cats, have shown that there is considerable electrical activity in the visual system during REM sleep where sudden bursts known as spike discharges have been recorded from within the brain. Such spikes have been found during rapid eye movements in the pontine reticular formation of the brain stem, and in two centers of brain that form relay depots for impulses as they travel from the eyes and optic nerves toward the back of the cortex and the occipital region involved in vision (Jouvet; Michel et al., 1964).

The eyes are, of course, ordinarily important in maintaining physical balance, although much of our neural apparatus for adjusting balance depends upon the vestibular system leading from the ears. Here, too, in spite of the fact that our postural muscles lack tonus during sleep, neurons of the vestibular system show bursts of rapid discharge during the rapid eye movements of REM sleep (Bizzi et al., 1964).

Similar bursts of electrical activity have been observed in the visual cortex and in the eye muscle (Michel et al., 1964). This latter activity did not seem to originate in the retina or in the nerve receptors of the eye muscles, nor in the cortex as one might expect of an imagined vision. Even when extrinsic ocular muscles and eyeballs were removed, the pattern of discharges on the visual cortex and brain stem remained the same. By surgical cuts, it was shown that this discharge activity did not come from the cortex and descend to the brain stem level. Instead, it seemed to originate in the pons of the brain stem and spread toward the eye muscles and central pathways of the visual system.

During REM sleep distinctive discharge patterns can be seen in another part of the visual system, the lateral geniculate. The altered firing patterns of these cells do not seem to come from the retina and its nerve routes, but possibly come upwards from the pontine reticular formation in the brain stem (Bizzi, 1965). This is an unexpected link in the brain network that may contribute to the visual imagery of dreaming.

Close readings of electrical potential changes in the eye muscles during REM sleep show a more rapid and chaotic activity than any seen in wakefulness, suggesting that dream imagery would have to be incoherent to produce such a scanning pattern. This is, of course, possible. We may write the connective scenario of dreams after the hodgepodge of images. One likely explanation suggested by the data may be that the eye movements are the result of "electrical" storms generated within the brain during dreaming and sweeping through portions of the visual system, bearing indirect relation to the visual imagery.

Kittens have been reared in total darkness, yet have shown rapid eye movements during sleep (Fishbein et al., 1965). Monkeys have been raised with contact lenses permitting some light, but no patterned vision, and they, too, show rapid eye movements in sleep (Berger and Meier, 1965). It has been observed that pupil dilations occur during the REM periods, phasically, but these occur in blinded cats as well as normal cats (Berlucchi et al., 1964), and may represent excitation that is not directly related to dream imagery.

Many facial muscles are spasmodically activated during dreaming. This is the time when babies suck or smile, when the cat's whiskers twitch. It is the time when people usually grind their teeth. A tree of nerves known as the trigeminal nerve branches to many facial muscles, including the masseters whose contractions result in teeth grinding. The motor nucleus, the root of this cranial nerve, is very near to a brain stem nucleus that emits great bursts of electrical activity during REM periods and perhaps transmits its excitation to these facial muscles.

If dreams are perplexing and strange, it is clearly a most strange state we are in as we dream. Our eyes move, we twitch, we may talk or utter sounds, we breathe shallowly and irregularly, our heart rate fluctuates, erections occur, and at the same time muscle tonus is very low and we are virtually paralyzed for short periods, often showing no knee reflex (Dement, 1965), while portions of our brain seem to be suddenly swept with storms of sudden, brief activity. What curious organization of the nervous system could be responsible for such an implausible interval in existence? Why might a brain that wakes and rests fall into these cycles of bizarre activity? What function could such a state serve in the survival of creatures as complex as man and as primitive as an opossum? How does this dreaming brain appear to behave?

Similarities to the Waking Brain

Probably the most striking thing about the dreaming brain is its resemblance to the waking brain as judged by some of its brain wave patterns. The brain is by no means precisely like the awake brain during REM periods, but it is quite different in its behavior from the brain during all other sleep. A truly enormous number of studies have emphasized this point; a good portion of these researches have compared evoked potentials from a brain site during waking and several phases of sleep. In this procedure a sound, a light, a touch, or some other stimulus is repeated and the brain's reaction is recorded in the instantaneous EEG pattern. This EEG response is minutely analyzed and each wave compared for size, duration, shape, and latency. Two kinds of findings of especial interest have emerged from this method. One is illustrated by readings from the scalp of human volunteers who received mild wrist shock. During waking and stage 1 REM sleep the EEG response is similar in shape, etc., close yet not identical. The segment of this response thought to represent the integrative areas of the brain that transform sensory impulses into feeling begins to arrive much more slowly from stage 1 sleep into stage 4. This suggests that the quality of mentation, somewhat akin in waking and REM, must change considerably during deep sleep (Allison, 1964, 1965; Rosner et al., 1963).

A second, seemingly paradoxical finding has been reported by Rosner and a number of investigators—essentially that sensory stimulation evokes more of a response during deep sleep than during waking or REM. Dr. Hernandez-Peon and his associates in Mexico City demonstrated this odd fact and suggested an explanation (Hernandez-Peon, 1965). During one study of cats, they recorded the electrical potential changes from the fifth sensory nucleus, a point where a nerve fiber bearing tactile impulses from the skin finally enters the brain. They touched the cat lightly on the face. During waking, this touch evoked only a small potential in response, suggesting that sensory stimulation was somehow being screened out. During REM sleep the potential was small, as well. But during deep slow-wave sleep the brain response was exceedingly large, suggesting that any filtering system must be virtually inoperative. Sensory inflow appeared to be heavily censored during wakefulness and dreaming sleep. Other studies suggest that some of this filtering is accomplished at the periphery.

Parallel studies performed during the late 1950's indicated that this censorship might be an essential ingredient of focused attention. Hernandez-Peon, recording from electrodes implanted in the optic radiations of patients undergoing diagnoses for brain surgery, had discovered that the EEGs showed a large potential when a light was flashed in their eyes at an idle moment, but that this potential was considerably diminished if the patient happened to be conversing when the light flashed. The potential declined similarly when the patient did a mental arithmetic problem or tried to recall a past event in his life. It looked as though a subcortical inhibiting mechanism were at work protecting the individual from irrelevant sensory inflow during moments of concentration, thus preventing a chaos of incoming stimuli from sabotaging all focused behavior. During REM dreaming and waking such a protective filtering may guard our capacity for attention, and indeed, protect sleep.

This similarity between brain response in waking and the REM state has been exposed by studies of man and different animals, performed for different reasons by Evarts, Rosner, Rosenblith, Segundo, Williams and Adey, to mention only a few.

Similarities have also been seen in the spontaneous activity of brain cells recorded at a time when no external stimulus was applied. Dr. Edward Evarts of NIMH has recorded from monkeys the activity of single cells in the pyramidal tract, which bears messages from the cortex to the motor system. Some cells showed the greatest frequencies of discharge in waking, were diminished in REM sleep, and lowest in slow-wave sleep. These cells showed least variability in waking, but greatest fluctuation during REM sleep. Curiously enough, the wild discharge irregularities they offered during REM sleep resembled the pattern when the waking monkey moved, reached for food, or scratched himself. Evarts and his colleagues were among the first to demonstrate that brain cells do not simply become inactive during sleep, but that they discharge differently, some of them more rapidly and more often. Electrodes implanted in the visual cortex of cats showed that the cells of this area increased their activity during REM sleep, a finding that seems consonant with the visual hallucinations of dreaming.

The dreaming brain also seems to be hotter than the brain in other stages of sleep. Moreover, a correlation between the changing brain temperature and EEG amplitude has suggested that this amplitude may be an index of brain metabolism (Rechtschaffen et al., 1965). Thus, it would seem that high brain temperature, and low EEG amplitude imply a high rate of brain metabolism, and are an index to the liveliness of mental activity in sleep and waking. Once again, the dream state seems to resemble waking rather than the quiescent stages of sleep.

Yet another kind of probe into the brain has told of some great similarity between waking and REM sleep. Dr. Heinz Caspars of the University of Munster implanted rats with direct current electrodes. Ordinarily, neurophysiologists use alternating current electrodes. Roughly speaking, the DC potentials showed a pronounced positive shift during slow-wave sleep, but they showed a negative shift during REM sleep. DC shifts corresponding to the alternating phases of sleep have since been seen in rabbits (Kawamura and Sawyer, 1964). These all indicate striking similarities between brain responses, cell activities, and background state in waking and dreaming.

A Difference From the Waking Brain

One very striking difference between the brain's responses in sleep and waking has been noticed in the great bundle of nerve fibers that connects the two halves of our brains. All mammals essentially possess two brains, joined in the middle by fiber bundles, the major one being the corpus callosum that runs down the middle of the cortex. By severing these fibers it has been found that they play a significant role in telling the right side of the brain what the left has perceived or thought, a major integrating function. Neural cells of the cortex, associated with the corpus callosum, show intense activity during attentive wakefulness, presumably coordinating the many activities within the brain. However, there is a progressive decrease of activity in these cells during sleep, and studies performed with implanted cats have shown minimal activity even during REM sleep. The activity of cells associated with this vast fiber system differ considerably in waking and sleep, and may suggest a more subtle distinction between the brain's capability in dreaming and waking (Berlucchi, 1965).

After a study of chimpanzees, whose sleep cycles and brain responses most closely resemble man's, Dr. W. R. Adey of UCLA has suggested that REM sleep is not deep unconsciousness but a state in which attention is concentrated internally when the creature is insensitive to peripheral stimulation—a state resembling those moments when an individual is so wrapped up in thought or in a book as to be virtually oblivious to the distractions around him. Although many neurophysiological studies and especially recent studies of chimpanzees emphasize great differences between the sleep mechanisms of man and those of

231

lower animals, it is interesting to note that many experimenters working with cats or other animals have come up with the same description of REM sleep as a state of inward concentration.

The Neuroanatomy of the REM State

The brain anatomy of the REM state, insofar as we can decipher the puzzle, has been exposed by a number of researchers. It has been explored brilliantly by Michel Jouvet and his associates in Lyon. Their research on cats, on accident victims with head injuries, on normal people, has led them to conclude that dreaming is a unique state, that two different neural systems must control sleep and the REM state. In a sense, they have postulated a dream-inducing center in the brain stem whose activation is associated with the many physiological changes seen in dreamers.

Occasionally an infant is born with only a brain stem, hydranencephalic. Because it has no regulatory mechanisms to keep it alive, such an infant usually dies very rapidly. If maintained artificially, however, this tragic creature, with only brain stem for a brain, shows EEGs and rapid eye movements like those of the REM state (Pierce et al., 1965).

Severe head injuries may cause regions of white matter to degenerate; this white matter consists of millions of tiny nerve fibers that connect one part of the brain with another. Thus a person who is decorticated in an accident is not devoid of his cortex, but the descending cable system enabling voluntary commands to reach the rest of the brain, and thus the body, are now destroyed. Accident victims, who on autopsy show that they were decorticate, may live for several years, bed-ridden, staring aimlessly, sleeping only for short intervals, unable to see, hear, or follow commands. Jouvet and his associates observed that such people, during sleep, showed every sign of being in a REM state but not slow-wave sleep. Slow-wave sleep seemed to require descending impulses from the cortex and was prevented by decortica-tion.

Other accident victims, observed over several months, seemed to be "unconscious" yet almost permanently awake. For short intervals they would appear to sleep, and this was always slow-wave sleep. There was great muscle activity dur-ing this time, and tonus very rarely disappeared; there was no sign of REM sleep. On autopsy it was clear that these people had been damaged at the lower part of the midbrain and in the brain stem pontine reticular formation. This corrob-orated laboratory experiments with cats—suggest-ing that the knob of neural tissue at the base of the brain, the pons, must regulate the REM state, and without its activity there would be no REM sleep (Jouvet, 1960, 1961, 1962).

Jouvet and his colleagues have performed in-numerable experiments upon cats to explore in a precise and refined manner the effects long seen in accident victims. By stages, they destroyed small areas of nerve fibers and watched what hap-pened to sleep. When they decorticated cats, the animals slept only in the REM phase and no longer showed the synchronous waves of deep sleep that seems to emanate down from the forebrain. Many people, in this laboratory and elsewhere, had induced sleep by stimulating hypnogenic areas in the forebrain.

When Jouvet and his colleagues stimulated the caudal pontine area of the brain stem, however, the cat would fall into a long interval of REM sleep. After many transections, they found that the caudal pontile nucleus must be crucial to REM sleep, for if it were destroyed, the animal no longer showed any of the characteristic signs in sleep.

When Jouvet destroyed the pontile triggering center, he found that the animals no longer had REM sleep. They were progressively dream deprived, and showed, in extreme, symptoms reminiscent of human volunteers in dream deprivation experiments. Many of the animals, for instance, became ravenously hungry and obese, and showed serious behavioral disturbances. Many of them showed behavior that seemed to be hallucinatory. These animals seemed to be the most telling examples of what severe and total REM deprivation could do, and of the importance of the pons to the dream state (Jouvet et al., 1960–65).

Recent findings confirming this observation have been phrased slightly differently (A. Camacho-Evangelista and Reinoso-Suarez, 1964). In the rostral part of the pons there must be structures responsible for activation, for when they are destroyed, there is synchronized rhythm in the brain. Within the pons itself, however, some lesions produce synchronization while others produce activation, depending upon location, indicating the complex duality of roles played by cells within this relatively small region.

In simple, perhaps oversimple, terms, there is a small region in the pontine brain stem area that is a part of a system that seems to generate arousal by its activity. Characteristically, it emanates low voltage, desynchronizing EEG patterns. These are the EEG patterns that are observed from the cortex and other regions during waking and REM sleep. However, when other areas of the brain above this region become active, they seem to generate the synchronous rhythms observed in deep sleep, in anesthesia, or coma.

The discovery that high activity within a brain stem nucleus seems to trigger the dream state may help to explain some of the peculiar bodily manifestations at this time. The pons lies close beneath the limbic system including the hypothalamus. In the human being, roughly speaking, this brain tissue resides just above the palate, above the roof of the mouth. This system, of which the hypothalamus is part, is associated with emotions and instinctual drives. Stimulations here can produce eating, drinking, rage, pleasure, abhorrence. By their anatomical connection, excitement from the nearby pontine region may spread into this area thus activating some of the responses (sucking in infants, erections) associated with the rudimentary elements needed for survival. As yet uncharted, these paths of excitation may be the physical foundations of drives expressed during dreaming.

Jouvet's work, augmented by the researches of other colleagues, has produced voluminous and elegant evidence that a very small area within the pons must trigger the electrical brainstorm we know as the REM dream state. Lesions within a tiny region of the pons would cancel out all paradoxical sleep in laboratory animals. Now, working within this minute region, Jouvet and his associates are beginning to elucidate some of the peculiar phenomena we have observed in the sleeper, the twitches, and sudden muscular contractions that occur in an interval otherwise characterized by body quiet and general muscular tonelessness. Within the caudal pons a small cluster of cells known as the nucleus coeruleus appears to generate the inhibition of muscular tone we see during REM sleep, an inhibition that prevents us from acting out dreams, or moving, even perhaps the most frightening inhibition, the frequent inability to scream out during a nightmare. When this tiny nucleus was destroyed by a lesion, the sleeping animal in paradoxical sleep moved a great deal, as if acting out a dream. His movements resemble sleepwalking, and indeed, this brain region may hold one of the keys to the mysterious phenomena of somnambulism. Although muscle inhibition no longer occurred when this nucleus was damaged, the phasic twitches—of the pupils of the eyes, of the whiskers, etc.—remained as usual.

Is the REM State Part of Sleep?

There is voluminous evidence that the dream state, whether it be known as activated, paradoxical, or simply REM sleep, is a state that differs considerably from the rest of sleep. Jouvet and others have suggested that it may be a totally different state, quite unlike what we usually consider sleep. Moreover, an impressive amount of evidence has been summoned to indicate that this peculiar second state of sleep is regulated by centers in the pons, invoking a quite different set of brain mechanisms and consequences than one finds in slow-wave sleep. This has been a strong and appealing hypothesis, and a very fruitful one, for it has generated an enormous amount of experimental work, which in turn has begun to illuminate some of the peculiarities of REM sleep. It is not, however, the only theory that attempts to explain REM state, and other investigators have not made up their minds that slow-wave sleep and the REM state are totally different states, subserved by two separate neural mechanisms. It is not at all surprising to find controversy about this issue, for the science is young, the explorations recent, and the brain is noted for its complexity and diffusion of functions. Thus, debate over the autonomy of neural mechanisms governing the REM state may continue unresolved, for some time.

One aspect of the debate revolves around the differences between higher mammals and man, and findings that suggest that structures far forward in the brain, the amygdala, may play a significant role in regulating the time we spend in each phase of sleep (Adey et al., 1963; Reite et al., 1964; Rhodes et al., 1965). In cats, during the activated phase of sleep, the hippocampus shows a pronounced theta rhythm, and very slight electrical stimulation to the hippocampal region will invoke the activated phase of sleep (Brown and Shryne, 1964). It has been suggested that the brain stem may exert a less potent influence in higher mammals and man, and the cooperation of phylogenetically newer and more cortical brain areas may be important to the REM dream state. Indeed, it has been suggested that the REM state may be a kind of rebound activity, interrupting long periods of cortical quiescence and general sensory isolation.

Many people have speculated that the phases of sleep are the outward signs of a feed back mechanism, in which the nervous system periodically "attempts" to wake up, increasingly often toward morning, yet before it is time for the sleep mechanisms to relinquish their dominance. Although no one has ever succeeded in finding that the body generates a hypnotoxin during wakefulness that triggers sleep and is used up in sleep, many people feel that sleep may be generated biochemically and that its alternating phases may represent a neurochemical feedback system.

Another comprehensive attempt to explain the REM state and some of its properties has been offered by Hernandez-Peon, who with associates has mapped an extensive hypnogenic system, running from the forebrain and thalamus, into the limbic system, with a center in the cerebellum. At several points it may overlap with the arousal system. Hernandez-Peon postulates that the dream state is a peculiar organization of events within the sleep system, not independent of it. Future experiments may reveal whether these two points of view are in total disagreement.

By direct electrical and chemical brain stimulation it has been possible to induce sleep along a hypnogenic pathway, sleep differing in depth, immediacy, duration according to the point stimulated—slow-wave sleep and paradoxical sleep. The hypnogenic pathway is set into action by cholinergic chemicals, but the investigators have discovered that cells adjacent to it could be activated by noradrenalin and adrenergic compounds to produce arousal. Thus, they will explore the possibility that parts of the vigilance or arousal system may be coextensive with the sleep-inducing system, in parallel, so to speak. If hypnogenic cells' activity dominates, there may be sleep; if the other system dominates, wakefulness ensues. The relative excitation strength of these two systems may dictate our state of consciousness.

Excepting in abnormal people or animals severely REM deprived, the REM state follows deep sleep. It occurs in sleep at a time when portions of the hypnogenic system hold the balance and inhibit the arousal system. Balance as conceived within the brain is not absolute any more than the balance of contending armies or of contending athletic teams who may shift in their gains and losses without any change in the overall score. Within the domain of hypnogenic dominance, regions associated with the vigilance system, among them centers in the pons, may periodically become activated as a part of an organization in which dreaming occurs and cells associated with awareness also become stimulated. Exactly what causes internal consciousness, without waking, nobody can say without further experimentation.

Neural links have been demonstrated, however, connecting peripheral muscle systems, the autonomic and endocrine systems, with regions of the hypothalamus and hippocampal and amygdala structures forward in the brain, regions that interact with the cortex. These numerous researches, mapping the way impulses travel through portions of the brain, have begun to suggest relationships between the peculiar state in which our closed circuit television experience of dreaming may be related to the physiological signs of muscle spasms, eye movements, heart and respiration changes (Feldman; Petsche; Yokota; Parmeggiani).

The chief EEG signal of the REM phase of sleep in man is a very fast, desynchronized rhythm, containing as one portion a theta activity, accompanied by rapid activity from the cortex, a pattern seen most clearly in cats and other animals in which there has been access to the hippocampus. This slow theta activity emanates from the hippocampus, a region of the brain that has been found to be intimately related to memory and emotional function. The universal example of its presumed role has been the epileptic, in whom damage in this hippocampal area causes severe memory impairment. The presence of hippocampal theta in animals during adaptation to a new environment, during periods that might be interpreted as anxious and fearful, suggests that these may be intervals in which the animal is incapable of taking in too much outside information. Hippocampal theta during waking shows continuous changes. During sleep, however, it has the appearance of a rhythm that is cycling, emanating occasionally to other portions of the brain, and maintaining a regular fast brain wave. This "circus movement" has been postulated by several experimenters (Brown and Shryne, 1964). It may be a fundamental property of the dreaming state, in which internal information, memory, and feeling seem to dominate the inward attention. Relationships have been observed between hippocampal theta activity, endocrine function (Sawyer et al., 1959), and autonomic and motor activity (Yokota and Fugimori, 1963, 1964). Others have shown that the influence exerted by the hippocampus during theta activity may be that of a feedback system, which opposes the influence of the reticular activating system in the sense of controlling the creature's reactivity to the outside world (Lena and Parmeggiani, 1964; Green and Arduini, 1954; Lissak et al., 1962). The relationship between the hippocampus and other brain regions crucial to the behaviors seen in dreaming has been shown by a number of studies (Parmeggiani, 1962; Buresova et al., 1962; Feldman, 1962; Manzoni and Parmeggiani, 1964; Jouvet, 1962; Brooks and Bizzi, 1963; Bizzi, 1965; Iwata and Snider, 1959). In essence the multitude of studies has shown that hippocampal theta rhythm is related to regions regulating emotion, autonomic, and somato-motor behaviors, and that these hippocampal rhythms may indeed be spreading from motivational areas in the hypothalamus and may be related to neural rhythms there (Petsche et al., 1962; von Euler and Green, 1960; Corazza and Parmeggiani, 1961).

Although the many interrelationships that have now been documented cannot yet be pieced together, the many elements of this puzzle are being collected througthout the world, so that we may soon begin to see the physical and neural components of the curious dream state. The function of the hippocampus in dreaming and in adaptation may indeed suggest a relationship between the dreaming individual, and the individual suffering from severe anxiety.

Animal Dreaming

Animal experimentation, on which we base so much of our understanding of man's brain, has always inspired a certain uneasiness. Animals show REM sleep, that we know, but do they dream as we do? Many people have thought so. Pet lovers watch a sleeping dog wag its tail, move its paws, wrinkle its nose, twitch its whiskers, or whimper, and imagine some internal world of action, pursuit, fear, pleasure. Is this creature experiencing some visual reenactment of its life? Until recently nobody had ever taught an animal to report "seeing things" in sleep, but this has now been done by Dr. Charles J. Vaughan of the University of Pittsburgh with rhesus monkeys and the procedure will be replicated.

While working on "sensory deprivation" phenomena as a gradute student with Drs. H. Braun and R. Patten, Vaughan helped to develop an elaborate training procedure. Its purpose was to ascertain whether "sensory deprivation" did actually produce neurophysiological changes and thus cause hallucinations in animals who, unlike human volunteers, would not be influenced by verbal suggestion. Rhesus monkeys were placed in a booth in which food and water were obtainable, but in which the environment was severely controlled; the background sound was a constant white noise like a waterfall, and the animals faced a ground glass screen. The monkeys were seated in a restraining chair with hands and feet resting on a bar holding shock electrodes. The monkeys were progressively adjusted to the situation and trained to press the bar rapidly every time an image appeared on the screen; otherwise, they were shocked on the foot. When they reliably responded to any kind of image on the screen by pressing the bar 3,000 times an hour, they were ready for a 74–96 hour period of sensory monotony.

In order to give them a constant and nonpatterned visual field, they were fitted with corneal contact lenses made of plastic, and then the door of the booth was closed, and the observer could watch through the window as the monkey sat in isolation. Like the many human volunteers in such experiments, the monkeys fell asleep soon after the isolation began. During sleep they showed three characteristic kinds of eye movements, a slow-rolling movement and rapid conjugate movement, sometimes resembling those of a person rapidly scanning the narrow column of a newspaper.

During these rapid-eye-movement periods, the monkeys suddenly began pressing the bar at a frenetic pace, rapidly and regularly as in waking. Sometimes they also made facial grimaces, flared nostrils, breathed deeply, even barked as they pressed the bar. Presumably they were "seeing things" during these intervals of rapid eye movements and were avoiding the shock associated with images. After the isolation period was over, the monkeys were tested in the training situation to be sure that they still responded reliably to the projected images. The investigators had seen only one instance of bar-pressing during waking, so they had little data about hallucinations, but the evidence that monkeys experience visual images in sleep was very strong.

Further studies using EEG and polygraph recordings will be undertaken by others to corroborate this. Perhaps a next step—training monkeys to respond to particular images or to smells, for instance—may allow us to find out what a monkey dreams about. Although the question of animal dreaming has interested pet lovers, animal trainers, and idle spectators, it has real importance for psychology. We have learned very little about the interior fabric of consciousness in animals even though they are the prominent instruments of our explorations into our own behavior. Each demonstrated similarity between experimental animals and man will strengthen the applicability of research to humankind.

The importance of animal research in unravelling the secrets of the REM dream cycle cannot be overemphasized. To date, although there have been quite a few human studies, most of our neurophysiological evidence has come from examining the brain reactions of cats and a few other animals, including monkeys. The data from these studies have arrived rapidly in the course of a single decade, inspiring new hypotheses about the nature, organization, and purpose of the REM state. These animal studies have helped to delineate a phase in the existence of all men, all animals, that now looks even more exceptional, provocative, and anomalous than it may have 10 years ago, when attention cohered around the vivid dreaming that recurred periodically throughout the night. Is this a unique state, something we should designate as a third state of consciousness, unlike sleep or waking? Does the REM state serve some vital life function?

Surely, in all mammals sleep is distinguished by two alternating phases. The curious, recurring REM state is an interval of activation in parts of the central nervous system, a period that includes dreaming, changes in autonomic functions, brain temperature, blood chemicals, muscle tension. These many REM phenomena seem to be the consequence of an integrated neural mechanism, but why such a conglomeration of events during sleep? Is this the testimony of some mysterious function without which we would die?

By degrees, REM deprivation studies of man and animals have aimed to find out how vital REM sleep may be. If removed from a creature's repertoire would the loss be followed by progressive deterioration and death? Initial human studies suggested that psychological changes followed fast in the wake of REM deprivation. Later and longer studies sometimes failed to show up psychological deterioration. Experimenters have always been very cautious about pressing human volunteers, and whenever ominous signs of behavioral change appeared the study has been terminated. Although some cats have died after

26 days' deprivation, other cats have been pressed to very long periods of deprivation, as long as 70 consecutive days without causing death and often the behavioral consequences were less severe than expected.

A Limit to REM Compensation

In recent experiments by Jouvet and Dement, it has looked as if the nervous system may have a safety device after a certain limit of REM deprivation has been reached. One of the uniform effects in all dream deprivation studies is the aftermath, or recovery, in which the individual appears to be making up the lost REM time by spending a far larger proportion of his sleep in that phase, finally, in the course of many nights, compensating for the entire loss. This pattern of compensation suggested that REM sleep might be triggered by some natural chemical that was produced at a steady rate and used up during the REM period. It was assumed that the deprived subject must be paying off a biochemical debt. More recently, however, deprivation experiments with cats have suggested that there is a limit beyond which the compensatory REM sleep no longer increases.

Jouvet has deprived cats of paradoxical sleep by placing them on a stone surrounded by water so that the loss of muscle tone accompanying the onset of REM sleep would cause them to fall into the water and wake up. When removed from this perch and placed in a recording cage the animal would quickly fall sleep, and during the first 6 hours it was possible to see how much more REM sleep occurred than usual. After 24 hours there was a 45 percent increase. After 72 hours there would be a 60 percent increase, and even after 22 days there was never more than a 60 percent increase in those first 6 hours of uninhibited sleep. As previous studies with animals and man have indicated, not all of the recuperation occurs during a single stretch of unrestrained sleep. After 10 days of deprivation a cat may take 5 days to compensate, and after 20 deprivation days, he may take about 10 days.

Dement, pressing a group of 20 cats to long stretches of deprivation found that they, too, showed the same effect. Until 30 days they exhibited continuous increase of REM sleep in recovery. However, at about 30 days they seemed to have reached a plateau. Even after 70 consecutive days of REM loss they showed no increments in their compensation, and appeared to pay back about the same amount they did after 30 days. It appears that the loss of paradoxical sleep is never totally reimbursed. If this signifies the accumulation of a chemical in the brain, a chemical that normally triggers REM sleep in the pons, one might expect that the accumulation would lead to brain stem damage. Surely, after prolonged deprivation, as shown in Jouvet's laboratory, the cats have exhibited what might be called an extraordinarily strong need for the paradoxical sleep. Even under heavy narcosis, they will show paradoxical sleep. After these long deprivations, they have also shown episodes of behavior disorder, sleep trouble, and several have died.

Experiments in the Biochemistry of REM Sleep

What is happening within a person or animal

in whom this recurrent cycle has been prevented? Dement and Jouvet have hypothesized that the REM state is triggered by a biochemical mechanism, possibly a chemical that is used up during the activation of the brain during the REM state. When a cat no longer discharged this chemical, perhaps it accumulated until it reached such concentrations that it could pass through the brain-blood barrier. It might literally leak out of the central nervous system. This might explain why the deprived cats seemed to reach a limit beyond which they no longer reimbursed the REM sleep they had lost. If such a leak occurred, one might expect to detect the triggering chemical within the spinal fluid.

One method of ascertaining a change in spinal fluid would be to take the cerebrospinal fluid of a severely deprived animal, inject it into the spinal fluid of a normally rested animal, expecting that the recipient would show a sudden increase in REM sleep. This is the gist of a procedure that has been performed at Stanford University under the direction of Drs. Dement and Peter Henry following the pattern of transfer studies in pharmacology.

Fine catheters were implanted into the third ventricle and cysterna magna in donor and receiver cats. This enabled the experimenters to draw spinal fluid from one, and inject directly into the other. The receiver cat was scheduled so that his sleep and amount of REM time became relatively constant and measurable. The donor cat was dream-deprived until he began to show behavioral changes, either by constant awakenings or by being placed on a stone in a water bath. Then spinal fluid was transferred from the deprived cat's brain into the brain of the receiver cat. There are many difficulties in an experiment of this sort, and some of the cats reacted to the injections with fever. Nevertheless, after trying many pairs of cats the result looks positive. Receiver cats have been showing a distinct increase in their REM time after injections of spinal fluid from the deprived animal (Henry et al., 1965). The very fact that increased paradoxical sleep has has been obtained by transferring spinal fluid from deprived cats into rested ones, raises some interesting questions about the nature of the chemical and the nature of the brain.

A hint about the nature of a possible chemical has emerged from recent studies in Jouvet's laboratory. There, injections of a depressant, reserpine, totally suppressed paradoxical sleep, but the sleep phase would be restored by an injection of Dopa. Dopa is related to a familiar group of brain amines and is a precursor to noradrenalin (Matsumoto and Jouvet, M., 1964). Further experiments in this laboratory indicate that within a nucleus in the pons that appears to be responsible for one aspect of REM sleep phenomena, there are capillaries suggesting biochemical responsiveness, and that the region does respond to noradrenalin. Noradrenalin is sometimes referred to as a neutral stimulant and is released at many sites in the body and brain when an abrupt increase in survival activity is required, as when an individual is suddenly frightened and must get ready to run. Other investigators have postulated that noradrenalin and related neurochemicals may be the excitors in a balanced chemical code system, playing the role of activating brain regions that engender vigilance and arousal. If chemicals of the adrenalin family trigger REM sleep and accumulate during deprivation, one might anticipate signs of brain excitation in a deprived creature.

REM Deprivation and Brain Excitation

Recently Dement's laboratory has amassed indirect evidence about the brain state of the REM deprived animal, evidence that suggests a state of excitement in certain neural centers. A group of cats, whose sleep was scheduled by placing them on a treadmill for 16 hours a day, were permitted to sleep for 8 hours, and were awakened at the onset of each REM period, getting only about 5–20 minutes of REM sleep a day. It didn't matter whether they endured this routine for more than 30 days; even at 70 days, when permitted free and uninterrupted sleep, they never reimbursed more of their lost REM time than they did after 30 days. However, as severity of deprivation increased, it became almost palpable in their REM sleep, for these intervals grew exceedingly intense. The animals were seized with twitches that now appeared almost like great spasms. The REM temperature change in the brain of one deprived cat was three times larger than his usual temperature rise, during normal baseline REM periods.

In another study, after only 4–5 days of REM deprivation rats showed a greater susceptibility to electroconvulsive shock. More curious, perhaps, was their reaction after the shock seizure. They no longer showed the usual recovery cycle when left to sleep unrestrained. They appeared not to need compensatory REM sleep to the extent of the deprived but unshocked rats. Did electroshock affect the animals' brain processes so as to perform the same discharge as REM sleep? Is REM sleep, in effect, using up the elements of unusual brain excitation?

Electroshock therapy has always presented something of a mystery, and there is no good explanation of why it works for certain psychoses. Perhaps its calming function is analogous to that of REM sleep, and related to the same mechanism of reducing brain excitation. Dement, Gulevitch and their associates have begun to explore the effects of electroshock in patients and laboratory animals. Initial findings indicate that people show less REM sleep after shock treatment, suggesting again that electroconvulsive therapy performs some of the same functions as does the REM period.

Is REM sleep, then, an end result of a metabolic-neural cycle, one which is normally discharged during waking behavior, but which builds up periodically during the quiescence of sleep until it reaches a discharge threshold? Are the psychotics who benefit from shock therapy victims of an abnormal metabolism, in whom production is overabundant, or discharge inefficient so that metabolism outstrips the ability to maintain a balance within the central nervous system? If so, the narcoleptic syndrome, with its sudden plummeting out of wakefulness into a REM seizure, looks as if it might be one of nature's makeshifts, a mechanism by which the brain discharges overexcitation before psychosis can begin.

The term "excitation" is extremely general, but it is probably an efficient designation for the state that is observed during REM sleep, and enhanced by deprivation. Insofar as it can be defined, it has been defined by deprivation studies. During deprivation, for example, Jouvet has found that cats show a marked increase in heart rate that settles back to normal after recovery sleep. The electroconvulsive seizure threshold drops in deprived rats. The intensity of REM intervals increases. This may be related to increased number of eye movements seen in psychotic patients at certain periods by Feinberg and his associates. The dream deprivation literature probably contains many references to the intensity of REM recovery sleep, although most observers did not emphasize these signs because they were concentrating on the amount of REM recovery and other aspects of the procedure.

The intensity of a REM interval has intrigued investigators, who have suspected that there may be a relationship between the intensity of physiological events, and the intensity of the dream experience. There have been suggestions that violent, active dreams, heightened psychic activity occur at times when the density of eye movements is great, when there are sizable changes in respiration, etc. (Rechtschaffen et al., 1963; Snyder, 1963). A number of people have attempted to knit together data from brain research in order to explain how memories, thoughts, images and emotions, are built out of patterns of neural excitation into dream experience (Fair, 1963; Brown and Shryne,

1964; Hernandez-Peon, 1963–65). Although the attention of some investigators has turned toward the possible biochemical and neural mechanism of the REM state, disparate evidence again seems to point to the same expectation—if an individual is deprived of the releasing mechanism of the REM state he may eventually incur a penalty, perhaps creating transient symptoms like those of psychosis, and ultimately causing severe damage.

It is, of course, impossible to excerpt REM sleep from the life of an individual as if it were as discrete as a wart or appendix. Manipulations within the laboratory undoubtedly create some collateral stresses. Nonetheless, control subjects matched with deprived subjects, whether animal or human, have not reacted the same way to awakenings in other sleep.

The quality of the response to deprivation has been respecified by Dement, in recent studies of severely deprived cats. They have appeared to act as if their basic drives were intensified. Six out of twelve male cats exhibited abnormal and indiscriminate hypersexuality. When also deprived of food for several days, the REMless cats acted more eager and voracious than their controls. They seemed to be too ravenous for food to run a maze with a food reward. Although, in some sense, these cats seemed to show an exaggerated survival instinct, the various behaviors seen among REM deprived cats, if shown by a human being, would certainly place him in the security ward of a mental hospital (Dement, 1965).

The Biological Purpose of the REM State

The drive enhancement observed in REM deprived animals, the penile erections accompanying REM periods in humans, the sucking and mouthing of infants in REM sleep and other data, have suggested to several investigators that the REM state may serve its most important purpose for species survival, by activating the drive mechanisms of the embryo and developing young. Perhaps, as Roffwarg, Muzio, and Dement have suggested, the REM cycle in adults is an atavistic remnant, a brain activity whose main role was to gear the individual for survival by inciting the development of drive oriented behavior (Roffwarg et al., in press). The REM cycle does, nevertheless, persist throughout life. Even if we discover that it does not have a role in the biological survival of adults, it may promote survival in the human being in a psychological-behavioral fashion that would not be as necessary in subhuman species.

Human adaptation for survival requires all manner of behavioral niceties, and control over drive behavior is one of the paramount requirements. As basic drives are intensified, whether due to a general excitation from REM loss, metabolic abnormality, or unusual environmental constraints, an individual's defenses may begin to break down, possibly starting the concatenation of events that occur in the buildup to a psychotic episode. Even if REM loss were to do no more than raise a level of excitation so that a human being found himself losing his usual, carefully schooled grip on the expression of instincts and impulses, growing somewhat less repressed, his behavior would be maladaptive according to our social norms.

Summary

Questions about the possible relationship between the REM state and mental illness are taking on a new complexity as data accumulate. Explorations at many levels are beginning to delineate why each of us must spend regular nightly intervals in the dream state of REM; what is happening within our bodies and brains during this sojourn; what happens if we are deprived of this weird interval. These explorations are likely to prove invaluable in the understanding and treatment of mental illnesses, many of which are heralded and accompanied by a vicious cycle of sleep disorders. As new data arrive, the questions seem to multiply. Yet, in a sense the questions are not new. They have been rephrased. They speak to biochemical codes, metabolic cycles, neural pathways. Today speculations about the function of REM sleep, and its relationship to mental illness, may contain little of the traditional language of psychoanalysis, and references to surface similarities between dreams and hallucinations seem to have been upstaged by compelling physiological investigations. Nevertheless theories about the psychological content of dreams, their relevance to our behavior, and the role they play in our unconscious all stand to be elucidated by these physiological studies. Although information about biochemical or neural mechanisms are not addressed directly to the subjective adventures of dreaming, they describe the physical foundations of a psychological process. Unlikely as it would have seemed 10 years ago, these diverse researches are suggesting why we may discover certain pervasive themes expressing basic drives in the dreams of all men, and perhaps someday, in all animals.

Chapter VIII.
The Development of Infant Sleep

Almost all autobiographies begin as close to the beginning as the author can remember, with a drama performed in early childhood in which he participated, the story of his molding, the explanation of his metamorphosis. As we try to explain, more systematically, the forces that shape behavior, to understand the process of development, we find ourselves looking for the earliest cues in infancy. But the young infant says little about himself in behavior, and furthermore, he is almost always asleep—one reason why studies of infant development are now including examinations of sleep patterns. The EEG patterns of sleep reflect activity of different neural structures in the brain and these may tell a good deal about the maturation process of the brain.

The infant's sleep differs from an adult's in several important ways. During his first weeks of life a human infant is asleep two-thirds of the time. Unlike his parents, and often to their chagrin, he does not sleep for one long siege at night, but rather for short intervals, interspersed with brief periods of waking, a polyphasic pattern that is characteristic of all newborn mammals. This cycle slowly changes, and he remains awake for longer periods and begins to sleep as his parents do, usually to their great relief. From the beginning the infant has had them at a great disadvantage, for he would awaken them easily enough with a yowl for food or attention, but infants are not so easy to arouse from sleep. At first, and to a lesser degree as they mature, infants are very often in a REM stage of sleep.

A number of anatomical studies on animals and behavioral studies of human infants have been directed toward answering an important question: Can we relate the maturation of sleep patterns to the maturation of the nervous system and to learning? What neural apparatus is necessary before an infant can begin to stay awake for long periods and sleep for long periods? What does the decline of REM sleep tell about the maturation of the infant's brain? Can the brain wave patterns of infant sleep serve as the earliest indicators of normal or abnormal development?

Since the 1930's babies had been known to sleep for roughly 50 minutes at a time. Within this interval there are minutes of slow, even breathing and quiescence, alternating with periods of fast uneven breathing and restless motions. Dr. Eugene Aserinsky watched from the cradle side for a relationship between slow rolling eye movements and body motion, and in 1952, when he transposed his study to adults, discovered the rapid eye movements that

258

signify dreaming. On repeated inspection, infants also showed rapid jerky eye movements in sleep, and although we cannot imagine that the newborn infant experiences visual dreams, he appears to spend much of his sleep in the REM state (Dreyfus-Brisac et al.).

Judging from what we know now about the REM state, as it may emanate from activity within the brain stem, exciting nearby regions associated with drives and emotions in the limbic system, it might be called a primitive activity of a primitive brain. The sleep of high amplitude, synchronous waves seems to depend upon the cortex and higher regions of the brain, as we have learned from decoticate accident victims and transected cats who no longer show slow-wave sleep.

The Decline of REM Sleep With Age

The regions associated with REM sleep seem to develop long before the cortex in its many folds and convolutions. In the embryo, the nervous system begins from nothing more than a tube of neural tissue. At the tail, the tube begins to form the spinal cord. At the head, the tube bulges into a forebrain, a midbrain and a hindbrain, and slowly these rudimentary bulges enlarge and fold. Slowly the cerebral hemispheres form, and last of all, during childhood, the outer layers of the cerebral cortex acquire their final convolutions. The hindbrain and midbrain develop long before the cortex and before the elaborate fiber network of communications is established between the cortex and the rest of the brain. Can we infer something about the rate of cortical development in an infant by watching his sleep, particularly the decline of the primitive REM state?

Only recently a number of investigators have indicated that the REM state does decline in infants as they mature (Parmelee et al., 1961–65; Roffwarg et al., 1963). By observing the sleep of young infants at progressive stages of development, they have all noted that the proportion of REM sleep declines during the first months of life, a clue that may help the pediatrician to chart the maturation of a baby's central nervous system and diagnose such abnormalities as retardation or schizophrenia at a very early stage of life.

It is interesting to note that monkeys follow a similar course. A recent polygraph study of newborn and infant rhesus monkeys indicated that for the first 7 days of life, the infant sleeps more, and a large proportion is REM sleep. After this critical seventh day the proportion of REM declined although total sleep time remained relatively constant throughout the first year (Meier and Berger, 1965).

From sleep studies of people of different ages including a premature infant born 10 weeks early and an old woman of 100 years, we can see approximately how much of one's sleep is spent in the dream state as one moves through life's timetable. In an infant, 10 weeks premature, 80 percent of sleep was REM sleep, but this ratio dropped as the infant approached full term, and in infants arriving only 2–4 weeks early the percentage of REM had dropped to 58 percent, and was 50 percent in the full term neonate. By 5 weeks REM sleep occupied only 40 percent; by a year only 35 percent; by 2–3 years, it had dropped to 30 percent, and by 5 years, 20 percent. Throughout later childhood and early adolescence, according to the limited observations available, the REM state dropped slightly, and in early adulthood rose slightly, ranging between 20–24 percent, again beginning to decline after about age 45 to about 13 percent in some of the aged persons studied. This is a very approximate schedule of the proportion of REM sleep occurring at any given age, but it suggests a developmental pattern of neural activity that begins in the cradle and follows a regular curve throughout life (Fisher, 1965).

A normative study of infant sleep may tell whether the decline of REM sleep is so precisely correlated with age that it might be used as a measurement in infant diagnostics. Such a study, begun in the UCLA laboratory of Dr. A. H. Parmelee, will encompass systematic observation of 100 infants from birth into childhood. New techniques for recording heart rate, EEGs, muscle tone, temperature, and respiration now permit such measurements even on very young infants and the premature. Recordings are being taken within the hospital nursery as soon as it is safe and comfortable for the baby, who is also watched by two observers. Once they leave the nursery the infants will periodically sleep in a special recording bedroom where they can be accompanied by their mothers. Then, as soon as they are old enough, they will receive graded batteries of behavioral tests at regular intervals.

An initial study of 46 infants has indicated the progress of the shift from polyphasic sleep to a diurnal pattern. This shift toward nightly sleep occurs in infants by about 16 weeks, even though they spend no more than about 3 hours awake in any 24 hour period (Parmelee et al., 1964).

Initial studies of premature infants, who must complete their embryonic development outside the womb, are beginning to show us something about the brain activity of the maturing unborn. Very premature infants (born 10 weeks early) do not show an EEG pattern like that of the full term baby. They seem to alternate between one state of drowsiness and another, and to exist in the REM state predominately. By taking EEG tracings during a 12-hour period of sleep, one such infant was observed to spend 80 percent of his time in the REM state. Less premature infants (6 or 7 weeks early) spent only 67 percent of their time in REM and the full term infants about 50 percent. By 8 months of age, this percentage dropped to 24 percent.

This steady and rapid decline in REM time was noted by Dement, Roffwarg, and Fisher, in studies conducted by watching the eye movements of infants in the nurseries of Chicago Lying In and Columbia Presbyterian Hospitals. Infants of many mammal species also have been observed to spend less sleeping time in the REM state as they matured. What might this decline of primitive activity mean in the anatomy of the developing infant brain? Could it mean that the growing tentacles of the cortex are beginning to gain greater contact and control, and that the brain stem is diminishing in its dominance?

Cortical Development in Kittens

Some suggestive answers have been coming from the anatomical and behavioral studies of Drs. Arnold and Madge Scheibel at UCLA. They have been engaged in a long program of studies of kitten development, seeking the concomitants of gross behavioral maturation within the growing neural fibers of the brain. The newborn kitten has a messy EEG and it is hard to tell whether the creature sleeps or wakes. As it grows the EEG begins to show differentiation, corresponding with the growth of nerve fibers. Dendrites, receptor fibers of the cortex, can be stained conveniently, although the transmitter fibers, axons, cannot. Consequently, the dendrites or receivers have been the first to be studied.

The dendrites of the newborn kitten are very simple. They resemble plants with a single smooth root, incapable of multiple contacts with other cells. Within the first days of life these dendrites begin to sprout long strands in many directions, giving more surface for contact with other nerve cells. These fine rootlike spines grow more numerous and dense with age, putting out side excursions that may indicate multiplying contacts between the cortex and reticular system.

The Scheibels have used pairs of litter-mates in their studies, recording the behavior and EEG measures of one kitten and simultaneously studying the brain tissue of its littermate. Within the same litter they found that kittens varied con-

siderably in their rate of maturation. Characteristically, the slow kittens were born with smoother
brains, an archaic and unarticulated cortex. The
kittens who showed rapid development were often
born with a more mature cortex, and their EEG
patterns differed commensurately. The smooth-
brained kittens gave slower rhythms in waking
and showed the spindling of sleep much later than
the kittens with convoluted cortex, maturer brains.
This difference appeared in behavior as well. The
more mature kittens snuggled against their mother
and sought milk in a purposive fashion.

Roughly, as they observed kittens through the
first 6 months of life, the Scheibels began to see
EEG progressions that differentiated the "normal" kittens from those with developmental disturbances. At what stage in a kitten's life, or in
a human infant's life, does brain development permit some voluntary control over waking? Is this
a stage at which infants begin to shift to the
diurnal sleep pattern of their parents? The Scheibels have performed conditioning experiments to
determine at what age a kitten might learn to
awaken. Kittens were trained to wake up and
reach for a bottle of milk when their names were
called.

The first kitten was tested by calling his name
during slow-wave sleep when he was 68 days old.
His EEG gave no sign of arousal. When the test
was repeated at 117 days of age, the kitten's brain
wave pattern quickly showed the desynchronized
pattern of arousal, and he got up and began to suck
at the nipple. However, he gave no sign of
arousal when a meaningless name, one he had

never heard before, was called. However, between about 9 weeks of age and about 16 weeks, the kitten had acquired the capacity to control his awakening.

The brain maturation of the kitten was clocked in yet another way, by direct stimulation of the reticular formation, the arousal area of the brain. Kittens, implanted in the reticular area and other deep brain sites, were stimulated during sleep at different ages. Newborn kittens did not awaken to rapid pulses; they only awakened after slow stimulation to the reticular formation. Moreover, their EEG response to brain stem stimulation appeared to fatigue quickly. After two repeated stimulations had aroused it further stimulation failed to awaken the kitten. Similar behavior is seen among human infants, who do not arouse easily from sleep. The Scheibels have conjectured that the undeveloped enzyme systems of the new-born brain cannot supply the rudimentary neural contacts rapidly enough, and so after these nerve cells fire a few times, the supply of chemical transmitters may be exhausted. Lack of neurochemical supplies may explain why the infant can do what no adult can do—disregard repeated stimulation direct to the arousal centers of the reticular formation.

This rapid adaptation to stimulation, internal and external, is a talent that the infant loses with maturation, just as many of the sensitivities and talents of the human child are, like eidetic imagery, lost by adulthood. These seem to decline during the very process of maturation by which voluntary controls are gained. Experience, itself, appears to be the teacher in a very literal sense, for repeated experience appears to alter the brain tissue and make it more responsive.

Ordinarily, experience does not come by electrical stimulation of the brain, but this is a kind of artificial experience. Brain stimulation does cause observable changes in the brain tissue of the kitten. Neurons connect with each other by sprouting boutons at the ends of their axons. These boutons then contact the receptor fibers, or dendrites, of other neurons. After electrical stimulation in an area, these boutons swell in size, and enlargement that can be seen under the microscope. The engorging of these boutons may be an accumulation of fluid, perhaps trapped by increased sodium ions. Similarly, it is supposed that after repeated stimulation an axon will grow in size and in its capacity for transmitting neural messages. Until now, the impact of experience, or stimulation upon the size of these contact fibers and links has been seen only after the fact, by placing specimens of brain tissue under the microscope. Now, however, an exceedingly elaborate microscope system with powerful lighting may make it possible to look into a living cat's or monkey's brain and watch the brain cells change as the animal is stimulated by repeated touches, light flashes, or sounds. If the technical obstacles are not insurmountable it may be possible to see into the brain and watch it grow during experience.

Here we may begin to see the anatomical changes, the neural growth that underlies the changing EEG patterns and behavior of the infant animal. By inference we may begin to understand what we are now observing from the surface, as we study the EEG changes of developing human infants during sleep. Perhaps we can begin to track the connections sprouted in the growing brain between the cortical areas and the reticular formation as we see maturing activity in the reduction of REM sleep, and the growing dominance of slow-wave sleep as well as the shift from a polyphasic sleep resembling that of the cat toward the strong diurnal rhythm of adult man.

Diagnostic Possibilities

The gathering of normative data and the process of inference from animal studies to human development are both very slow and expensive, but there is reason to hope that they will be exceedingly useful in diagnostics and for an understanding of the integrity of nervous function in infancy. The common story of mental retardation and malfunction is a tragic one, in many cases because it is detected late in childhood development when remedies are less and less potent and more elaborate. What amounts to mental retardation in late childhood could sometimes be prevented by the detection of a simple yet ramifying defect, during babyhood, which sometimes amounts to poor visual control, hearing, or to an insufficient rate of development that ends up in leaving a person totally behind. If such defects can be spotted in earliest infancy remedies can be applied at the time when they will do the most good, for each successive stage of development hinges to some extent upon the last.

Unfortunately most abnormal behaviors are difficult to see in young infants. Many pediatricians have had the feeling that activity patterns in the newborn can suggest the maturation progress that will follow, but infant behavioral tests are inadequate. Psychiatrists have reported that extremely underactive or overactive infants seem possible candidates for childhood schizophrenia. When such babies are brought into clinics they often have a history of unusual sleep patterns. Either they seemed to sleep too much, or they harried their mothers by crying incessantly and sleeping briefly and irregularly. If the normative studies of Dr. Parmelee, and his colleagues prove fruitful, we may have another yardstick for normal development in the rate of REM decline. Infants who are very slow in this decline may suffer metabolic problems, causing what we now call retardation, in a form that can be ameliorated before there are lifelong ramifications.

Recent designs for extremely sensitive polygraph equipment may indeed permit Parmelee and his group to trace the development of infant sleep patterns back into the womb, allowing us to track the brain activity and physiological development of the unborn. REM activity may indeed represent the first concerted workings of the brain, a fundamental rhythm into which all later activity becomes knit, the first pulsing from which experience and growth will shape the growing psyche. The dream state of infants, while unlike the subjective and complex dream of the adult, may be the first expression of all the forces of survival provided by nature within the very cells of the primitive brain, the first practice of the funda-

mental instinct and drive centers—and their first
effector actions, seen as the sucking, smiling, kicking of REM sleep in the newly born.

Chapter IX.
The Meaning of Dreams

Unleashed from reason and detached from circumstance, the play of dreams is armed with terrible freedom. In all history and every recorded culture the mysterious and evanescent dream has been taken seriously. Strategic dream interpretations have altered the course of nations, as did Joseph with the fat kine and lean. Oracles dreamed the future. By pagan dream-rites the sick were healed. Lincoln's dream of death seemed a harbinger of his fate. American Indians enacted their dreams. During the reign of terror and superstition from the 12th through the 17th century, Western Europeans fought an international conspiracy of witches, and the seriousness of the dream was evident in the Malleus, guide and handbook to every judge of the Inquisition, at a time when dreams might mean burning. Dreams also inspired poetry in Coleridge, fiction in Robert Louis Stevenson, and Kekule, the organic chemist, is said to have deciphered the arrangement of atoms in the benzene ring by a dream of a snake eating its tail. The skillful man, said Emerson, reads his dreams for self-knowledge. Although dream books including codes for gamblers and advice on all aspects of practical life are abundant on newstands today, we tend to probe dreams for insight into the dreamer.

Dramatic, recurrent, universal to mankind, the dream is nevertheless an experience that people cannot share. The dream that is communicated is a memory from a sleeping state and the extent to which people must distort their dreams can be estimated by the imperfect court testimonies of witnesses who are attempting to report real events truthfully. There have been a number of attempts to ascertain the memory span for dreams. One, an initial study in the University of Chicago, by Drs. Edward Wolpert and Harry Trosman, showed that volunteers could remember dreams if awakened at the end of REM periods, but not several minutes later. Like the trace of the evanescent neutrino, the dream had to be captured at once or it evaporated.

A psychiatrist, whose patients were awakened in this laboratory, compared the immediate narratives with the patients' daytime recollection, and found that the morning versions were palpably different. Similar discrepancies were noted at the Institute for Dream Research in Miami, Fla., when monitored records from laboratory awakenings were compared with the written accounts by the same volunteers at home (Hall and Van de Castle, 1964.) The laboratory narratives were long and incoherent and less intense than the tightly organized home reports. There is no means of checking a dream report against a dream. However embroidered and shaped, however censored and skewed, we have only human recall for evidence. Until recently the dreams reported were usually the last of the night, just before awakening.

With today's electrical recording equipment it has been possible to sample the night's dreams. Customarily, volunteers will spend several nights in the laboratory, adjusting, while the investigator obtains EEG recordings that roughly indicate the individual's timing and spacing of dreams. He can predict when the subject will begin dreaming and approximately how long each dream period will last, awakening the subject toward the end of a segment.

Is there any relation between the several dreams of a night? Freud suspected that sequences of dreams elaborated the same motive, timidly at first and then more distinctly. Franz Alexander postulated that successive dreams were connected in pairs, and that a night's preoccupation was clarified by the repetition of a theme. Drs. Harry Trosman, Allan Rechtschaffen, William Offenkrantz, and Edward Wolpert studied 2 young men for 32 nights. Well over a hundred dreams were collected and analyzed, but only on one night did a subject have four dreams directly related in theme and content. The lack of continuity found in an earlier study by Dement and Wolpert did not outlaw the suggestion that a sustained emotional tone and recurrent items might pervade the night, and continuity was observed by Offenkrantz and Rechtschaffen (Offenkrantz and Rechtschaffen, 1963).

The possibility that dreams might have predictable and characteristic differences at different times of night was pursued by Dr. Paul P. Verdone, who found that the initial dreams seemed to revolve around current events, whereas dreams of childhood and past events occurred later, coinciding with the time of the person's lowest temperature. The longer a person had been asleep the more vivid and emotional his dream reports, the easier his recall. Then, after about 7 hours of sleep, the volunteers began once more dreaming of current elements in their lives. Work in progress at NIMH may illuminate the interesting correlation between low temperature and dreams of past events, and may determine whether the particularly vivid dreams are associated with time of day, time in bed, or body temperature (Verdone, 1965).

As a great many researchers have demonstrated, the REM dreams are not islands of imagination on a dark river of oblivion, for when people have been wakened between REM periods they have offered wisps, thoughts, fragments, and images. Perhaps these provide continuity among the REM dreams of the night. Drs. Allan Rechtschaffen, Gerald Vogel, and Gerald Shaikun have collected intermediate recollections from subjects and found that these non-REM elements resembling daydreams or imagistic thought may be interwoven into the REM content, demonstrating some continuity in the thematic fabric of the night. It is interesting that people talk throughout their night of sleep, and not only during REM dream (Rechtschaffen, Goodenough, and Shapiro, 1962). Studies of sleep talking indicate that it is a common occurrence and that it changes in tone, growing more expressive and emotional during REM periods.

Influencing Dream Content

Dreaming animals and people are incorrigibly wrapped up in their private worlds and are usually hard to awaken. Freud and others have postulated that the dream protects a person from awakening and that outside events may simply be incorporated in the dream. While working at the University of Chicago, Dement and Wolpert tested dreaming volunteers with lights, sounds, water. The stimulus was identifiably incorporated in only 20–60 percent of the dreams, but perhaps more of the dreams did interweave the outside disturbances in transmuted or symbolic form. (Dement and Wolpert, 1958). By objective assessment, however, Berger did find outside events highly incorporated in dreams (Berger, 1963).

The fact that we may not incorporate outside events into our dreams 100 percent of the time does not mean that we don't interweave these events some of the time. After applying heat or cold to sleeping subjects, investigators have obtained thermal references in only about 25 percent of the subsequent dreams. Because the incidence has been low in some well designed studies, there has been a tendency to feel that external events do not influence dream content very much. Similarly, bodily states such as hunger and thirst, have produced little impact on reported dreams (Dement and Wolpert, 1958). However, thirsty subjects, deprived of food and liquids, and then given a spicy meal before sleep, have referred to thirst to a degree that suggests a definite somatic influence on the actual dream content (Bokert, 1965).

There have been a number of attempts to manipulate the content of dreams. Dr. Johann Stoyva of Langley Porter Institute, San Francisco, assigned several volunteers dream topics by posthypnotic suggestion. When awakened and asked their dreams, only one or two dreams would contain these preassigned elements, which were instructions to dream of climbing a tree, etc. The notable effect, even with a well seasoned laboratory volunteer, was a reduction in the amount of dreaming (Stoyva, 1962).

Manipulations of dreaming behavior have interested many researchers, for individuals differ greatly in their responsiveness, perhaps indicating far-reaching constitutional and psychological endowments that would be useful to define. In studies already cited, some volunteers were able to hear and remember tape-recorded numbers while dreaming, sometimes incorporating them into their dreams; others could be motivated to press switches when entering a dream period or respond to signals. Rechtschaffen, at the University of Chicago, has paid volunteers to increase or decrease their amount of dreaming with a small effect on the amount of time spent in REM. (Rechtschaffen and Verdone, 1964). In each instance one might expect that individuals divide sharply in their responsiveness. Dr. Martin Orne, and his associates at the Institute of the Pennsylvania Hospital, have been conducting a program of studies on hypnosis, and in a recent pilot study find that deeply hypnotizable subjects can act upon suggestions delivered during dream periods, whereas less hypnotizable people will not follow sleep instruction. During sleep, with no prior hypnotic suggestion, volunteers were told that the word "pillow" would make the pillow seem uncomfortable and they should move it; the word "itch" would cause their noses to itch until they scratched. When the instructions came during REM dreaming, the deeply hypnotizable subjects did indeed move their pillows and scratch their noses. The others either gave no response or awakened. This difference in suggestibility, evident in sleep and waking, is a curious phenomenon (Cobb et al., 1965). People differ quite as sharply in their ability to remember dreams.

Dream Recall

Ten years ago it was possible for a person who remembered dreaming every night to look with pity on the impoverished soul whose nights were devoid of imagination—the person who said, "I never dream." Now it seems clear that we all dream about the same amount, every night. Why do some people not remember? There have been many speculations on this point. Patients in analysis, motivated by questioning, begin to remember dreams. Personality differences have been discovered in which introspective people have seemed to recall dreaming most easily. The question of dream recall prodded Drs. Donald Goodenough, Arthur Shapiro, and their associates at the New York Downstate Medical Center into a long program of studies. Many factors were at play. For instance, the faster a person awakened the more fully he would describe a dream, so the mode of awakening mattered (Shapiro et al., 1963). However, individuals differed in the amount of noise that would awaken them. Those who normally remembered dreaming at home would awaken quickly in the laboratory, after a horrendous 80 decibel blast, and recite a rich dream narrative. People who rarely remembered dreaming at home, when aroused into wakefulness often thought they had been awake and thinking the whole time. One young man delivered a bizarre narrative about sitting in class popping pennies into a vending machine and striking oil—yet asserted he was thinking. He could control his dream, he explained, in the manner of a daydream, and he was aware of sounds in the room, such as the air conditioner. This kind of explanation and a wealth of other data suggest that there might be distinct physiological differences; some people dreaming at a lighter than normal level of sleep and thinking themselves awake, while others dream in a deeper than normal stage of sleep and lose their dreams in the long process of awakening. But there seems to be another kind of forgetting as well, possibly repression (Shapiro et al., 1964; Goodenough et al.).

Dream Intensity

Some guidelines have emerged during the last few years for estimating the emotionality of a dream from physiological measures. Dr. Frederick Snyder of NIMH and others have correlated physiological changes with dream content. One sign that suggests an intense dream is highly irregular respiration, like the breathing of a person in terrible anxiety or impatience. Dr. Charles Fisher of Mount Sinai Hospital has shown that penile erections accompany almost all dreaming periods in males, from birth on, and dreams that are not accompanied by erection or which have sudden detumescence appear to be dreams of terrible anxiety, of violence and body mutilation. Some thousands of nights have now been dreamed away in sleep laboratories, and many investigators have observed physical symptoms that suggested an intense dream, only to find out when they awakened the person that he did not remember, or only gave a vague and bland story.

Stimulation Before Sleep

Investigators at the New York Downstate Medical center are currently watching the physiological symptoms and EEG configurations of volunteers who have been exposed to films before sleep. On one night there is a pleasant, neutral travelog. On other nights there is either an anthropological documentary showing birth or initiation rites, both quite disturbing. In a preliminary study of 10 people, Drs. Herman A. Witkin and Helen B. Lewis found evidence that the elements of the presleep film were identifiably incorporated into the dreams of that night. By interview techniques and prior clinical information, the investigators have been able to connect the way the person dreamed about the material with significant events in his personal life. The subjects were transit workers, telephone engineers, bakers, airplane factory workers, and others who normally sleep during the day, and who had not been exposed to theories of psychology. Further studies using these films may discriminate between those people whose inability to recall dreams is related to physiology, and those who cannot remember disturbing experiences.

Many people have wondered whether a film seen just before sleep has an influence on one's dreams. Many parents have asked themselves this question as their small children gave rapt attention to a TV drama of monsters, or crime and violence, just before bedtime. In studies of the impact of mass media on children, some social scientists have postulated a direct influence on behavior. Dr. David Foulkes, when at the University of Chicago, sought another approach and looked for the influence of presleep stimuli on dreams. From its roots in a sociological interest, the study then took on quite an independent aspect. Adult volunteers watched two different films on two separate nights before retiring in the laboratory. These were network telecasts, one a typical western, the other a romantic comedy. By sifting the dreams for incorporation of the previous TV material, the investigator found direct influence in about 5 percent of the dreams. However, when he analyzed the emotional qualities of the dreams he found that the dreams following the western were far more vivid, imaginative, and highly charged than the dreams following the comedy. The results of this study do not conflict with the Downstate study, for the investigators used the kind of films a person might normally watch before bedtime. Witkin and Lewis employed traumatic and bloody films among theirs and were particularly interested in the metaphors by which an individual might transform material. For instance, a dream of taking cake from a bag appeared to be easily connected to the birth film the subject had seen a few hours earlier.

We know a great deal more about dreaming today than we did in Freud's time. We know more about the amount of dreaming in individuals of specified age, physiological changes that occur at the same time, the effects of drugs, some of the neurophysiological events. We can evoke behavior in dreaming and compare responsiveness and recall. We find that recall differs as the night wears on, improving toward morning. We may soon understand the biochemistry that triggers dreaming. All of our observations about the need to dream, the intensity of dreams, and how their incidence varies with illness are bound to be refined. But the meaning of dreams?

Grand and confident theories become more difficult to compose as the data accumulate, for today's theories require predictability, demonstrations that the relationships between dream and dreamer are not subject to the varying interpretations of investigators. Many of the dream reports obtained in the laboratories over the last 10 years differ from the types of dreams analyzed by Freud and others, yet many investigators feel that some of those early intuitive analyses were, in some sense, true. What beast is loosed at night from the cage of civilization to stalk through stark and perplexing dramas, perhaps cloaked in innocuous symbolism? How are these figments related to the day past, to the core of the personality, or to random noises in the bedroom? Does an obsessional nightmare relate to neurosis or physiological changes, are there dreams characteristic of health, and dreams bespeaking illness? These are important questions, and the modern dream hunter is equipped with new tools for exploring, but the dream reports are still memories and we do not yet have methods of checking the speaker's veracity from outside.

Classifying Dreams

Some years ago, before the advent of electronically tracked dreaming, some of these questions were attacked very differently—with methods a sociologist might use to classify the attitudes of people toward a sensitive issue such as birth control. Here, hopefully, statistics might be used on a large sample of questionnaires to filter out the small lies and obfuscations of individuals and reveal the general attitudes of people in different socioeconomic or regional groups. By amassing a truly enormous number of dream reports and applying statistical analyses, the Dream Research Institute of Miami, Fla., has been finding out the general kinds of dream content that typify certain groups of people: normal college youngsters, the physically ill, mentally ill, the aged, and people of particular ethnic groups.

The institute, founded and directed by Dr. Calvin Hall, is probably the largest repository of dream narratives in the world, its files containing some 30,000 dreams. Among these are 5,000 dreams collected from other countries and cultures, from Australians, Peruvians, Nigerians, Mexicans, and many others. Many of these dreams have been broken down into components, classified, and subjected to statistical procedures. If this method can render the distinctive dream patterns of a specific culture or distinguish between the mentally ill and the healthy, a dream report may become a diagnostic aid. Among other things, it may help a doctor foresee an impending mental breakdown, the onset of an acute episode, suicidal tendencies. It may provide us with useful insight into other cultures and in the differences in outlook between the sexes (Hall, 1951–65).

This empirical evaluation of dream content is based on a systematic categorization of each element or event. Dr. Hall and his associates have first classified items that occur most frequently: the kinds of characters that appear in dreams and their relationship to the dreamer, the setting, the objects, the dreamer's emotions, lucky or unfortunate events. Out of these analyses, they have developed manuals that might be used by a therapist, for instance, in analyzing a patient's dreams and judging whether these included more than a normal number of fearful events. Although this large scale normative study is still in progress, the manuals offer some guides for judgment by citing the distribution of the categories of dream events for specific populations. For instance, an analysis of 1,182 dreams reported by young men and women suggested that about 2 out of 5 dreams are fearful, often containing a sequence in which the dreamer is pursued. A similar assay implied that for every dream of good fortune, a person may have seven dreams of misfortune. The dreamer is more often the victim than beneficiary. Questionnaires filled out by students who contributed dreams indicated that they felt only about a quarter of their dreams were pleasant.

An analysis of 7,000 dreams shows up one notable difference between men and women. Men tend to dream about men, in general, but women dream equally of men and women (Hall and Domhoff, 1963).

A recent study of the dreams of 60 nurses suggests that women's physiological cycles may influence their dreams. A tentative assay of dreams before and during menstruation shows that women may dream of waiting for something, a bus, or train, during the premenstrual period, whereas dreams of destruction seem to occur during the first days of the cycle.

The institute's new sleep laboratory is unusual in the sense that it is located in a residential house and has little of the laboratory aura. Here, while attempting to obtain a representative dream sample from 25 healthy young unmarried men, the investigators hope to detect and correct the kinds of censorship and bias that have entered the dream reports collected outside the laboratory. As this empirical work continues on a grand scale, people continue to ask what do dreams mean. Are they wishes, unspoken or unadmitted by day? Are they a safety valve? Does unemotional, toneless dreaming indicate schizophrenia? Does one solve "problems" in dreams?

The task of interpreting dreams has grown no

smaller now that we can clock them, collect more of them, try to manipulate them. Today's accumulation of data has instigated a few very tentative speculations, for dreams, their images, sensations, emotions, are physically part of us, and the blue rhinoceros that stalks the salon of our dream reveals something of our nature. The images must come from somewhere.

Speculations About the Neural Basis for Dreams

Some investigators have speculated that they are made up of memories and are activated in the hippocampus, a neural formation that curls across the center of the brain like two horseshoes joined at the middle and curving outward toward the temples, ending in the amygdala. This region has been thought to act as a clearinghouse for memory, a stage before memories are filed for storage. Lesions of the hippocampus or amygdala will cause a loss of short-term memory. During the EEG phase that corresponds to the dream period, animal studies have shown bursts of rhythmic activity from the hippocampus—theta activity that spreads to a part of the brain that participates in awareness or attention. Perhaps this is the episode we call a dream. However, a simple kaleidoscope of images, memories, thoughts, would not explain the cold sweat of terror we suffer in a nightmare or the pleasurable involvement we sometimes experience. It would not explain why inconsistent images, the trivial intermixed with the momentous, appear to have some meaning we cannot explain. One very tentative explanation has been offered. In a word, it says that motivational centers within the brain are activated during dreaming and that these centers may structure our dreams. This is a familiar hypothesis. It was suggested by Freud in evolving a theory about the latent content of dreams.

Today, an anatomical hypothesis has been phrased by Dr. Raul Hernandez-Peon, and while it is emphatically tentative, it suggests a neural background for the significance of dreams, indeed perhaps explaining man's centuries of profound interest in dream symbols. A hypnogenic system extending from the front of the brain toward the spinal cord overlaps with a portion of the hypothalamus where stimulation evokes signs of pleasure—a center, one might say, for positive reinforcement and a positive component of motivation. Reactions of abhorrence have also been produced by stimulating another area in the hypothalamus, a center, roughly speaking, of punishment or negative reinforcement. Motivation, as we think of it, may be based on the sensations of pleasure or punishment attaching to certain acts or impulses. Pleasure or pain can be evoked by directly stimulating the brain, but like sleep and wakefulness, they are induced by stimulation from the outside world, by monotony, or sudden noises, that send their impulses up the spinal cord. Similarly, they can be induced, like voluntary sleep or waking, by impulses descending from the cortex, internally generated. It is quite plausible to think of this motivational system as active during sleep, and if so, it might be the editor, the shaping power behind our dreams. During our wakeful hours, especially in youth, we learn to suppress the behaviors and even thoughts for which we are usually punished. By maturity, we hardly pay attention to this constant suppression of antisocial impulses.

In waking life, when the vigilance system is active and dominant, our neural apparatus is energetically holding down these punished impulses. The fact that a region of negative reinforcement lies close to the arousal system gives some encouragement to this conjecture. During sleep, however, this very system that inhibits our punished impulses may be suppressed, itself by the activity of the hypnogenic system. Are repressed impulses now released in a manner resembling the release that comes with certain depressants like alcohol or anesthesias? If this be the case, the punished impulses could now emerge and place their positive or negative weight upon the welter of images that have been activated in this dreaming state of sleep. It is unnecessary to belabor the point that the most punished impulses of the child are those behaviors and curiosities directed by basic drives. If these are the suppressed factors that structure the otherwise incomprehensible mélange of dream material—they are indeed the elements of latent dream content, phrased somewhat differently by Freud.

This is a complicated speculation and built upon an enormous amount of anatomical and behavioral data. Although it may be unfair to cite the hypothesis so simply, it may indicate the new threshold over which dream interpretation—the question of meaning—may be moving. Neurophysiologists are beginning to suggest that dreams may be shaped by drives in an organization that brain research may soon begin to elucidate. A dream is a psychological phenomenon. It cannot be understood by physics. The act of dreaming, however, is both a psychological and a physical process, determined by our structure and the learning imposed upon our very cells.

Drive Mechanisms in REM

Freud might be privately amused to see the implications of some recent research. The intensive sleep studies of Dr. Charles Fisher at Mount Sinai Hospital in New York, suggest that the strong sexual motivation underlying dreams, as Freud saw them, might be even stronger than Freud supposed. Preceding every REM period, from infancy onward, males have penile erections. This does not mean they have overtly sexual dreams; indeed, what would such a dream be for an infant? Sexual activity, however, is part of our survival equipment and something toward which much learning must be applied, step by step. The REM sleep, in which erections occur, begins very early—in premature babies, perhaps in the womb. The function of REM activity, as Dement has suggested, may be that of a primitive core activity, a rhythm in the rudimentary brain into which all later motivation and learning interlocks, a first practice in the body learning that occurs with development. It is during this predominant phase of sleep that the infant first exercises his limbs, sucks, and smiles. This may represent a first practice in the effectors of the great drive forces for survival. Perhaps erections are involved in the body-brain learning process of the infant. Their existence suggests that sexual drive mechanisms develop from the start and are subject to influence by very early training. The function of such drive discharge in adult sleep is unexplained and could be purely vestigial. But in adults, they are connected with dream content. The interesting dream is the exception, the REM period that is not accompanied by erection or in which there is rapid detumescence. Data so far suggest that these are dreams of intense anxiety, often including body mutilation (Fisher et al., 1965).

The fact that there may be a strong connection between drives, dreams, and the covert symbolism of dreams does not give us a direct handle for the interpretation of specific dreams in relation to their dreamers, but it opens up new avenues of exploration that may not have seemed relevant to dream interpretation 10 years ago. By using tools now being developed in neurophysiological and physiological research, we now begin to look at the process by which dreams are formed. Here we may begin to find some of the complex but lawful processes by which living experience accrues in the brain and is transmuted into that most private experience, the dream. The anatomy of dreaming, as we may learn from animals, may divulge some of the roots of fantasy, revealing the way in which emotional learning encrusts event and sensory experience. From young children in various stages of maturation we may hope to learn about the impact of environment in its larger ramifications. The development of new analytic tools for reading brain wave rhythms and the accumulation of data allowing us to localize their sources may give us a kind of Geiger counter on the dreaming mind and its response to our manipulations from outside. Slowly we may learn how to disentangle the components of dreams. The findings and speculations mentioned here contribute to the disentangling. If the dream memory is to provide an understanding of an individual personality, to be useful in therapy or aid in diagnosis, we should be able to differentiate phsysiological cycles, from cultural idiosyncrasies, and from immediate events—seeing the pervasive style and shaping that is given to the dream by an individual. Since dreams are formed by physical processes, and since illness, mental or physical, presumably comes from alterations within our cells, it does not seem impossible that dreams might provide diagnosticians of the future with warning signals.

At present we have to rely upon intuitions and education sharpened by the mounting data. Science cannot encompass all life at one gulp, and life is the stuff dreams are built upon. Each of us in a private universe weaves together a myriad of experiences, important, and trivial— daily routine, learning, automatic responses of hunger or breathing, and moments as transient as an eyeblink. Embedded in the central nervous system, shaped by learning, these are the tools of conscious behavior. By day it all seems purposeful and real, the actuality confirmed by others, but the unsharable dream, for the most part, leaves no more impression on memory than the shadow of a leaf falling over a stone. Since we tend to recall the unusual, and for yet unexplained reasons do sometimes remember some figment from an implausible mirror-image world, we have throughout history concentrated upon these few gleanings and singled them out for the game of interpretation. Today, at least, we may sample the whole gamut, perhaps seeing them as the processes of all mammal minds and not interpreting them as a harbinger of external world events.

Chapter X.
Good Sleep and Poor

Every night of sleep is not the same, as we all subjectively know. One night may pass like a moment, from which we awaken serene, restored and vigorous; and yet the next night may seem fitful. We may arise soggily, as if from a long wrestling match. One's mood on awakening may be sunny one day and morbid the next. Each person varies somewhat from night to night. Worry may make sleep difficult, and sleep itself may seem light. Depression may make one sluggish or awaken one before dawn. Fever, alcohol, drugs, events, and a multitude of subtle unknowns play into the texture of a night's sleep and its dreams. Everyone seems to have a subjective feeling for the difference between a good night's sleep and a poor one, but for most people life contains a mixture.

Some people, on the other hand, complain that they are usually poor sleepers. Others know they sleep easily. Sleep studies have shown that people differ in the amount of time they spend dreaming, in their ability to do such things as press a switch during sleep, in their memory of dreams, indeed, as judged by the EEG record, some people have shown very unusual sleep patterns.

EEG Differences

Perhaps the first characterization of differences between people who sleep soundly and those who do not, emerged as a byproduct from an early test of Markovian chain analysis of the EEG sleep record. This is a mathematical technique for assessing the predictability of steps in a series. If a person were in stage 3 sleep, for instance, could one predict the probability that he would next move into stage 2 rather than stage 4? The raw material for this analysis came from eight volunteers, who spent four nights each in the laboratory. On analysis the Markov chains for their records separated them into two homogeneous groups, each with its chain of EEG changes. One chain characterized the four subjects who slept soundly through the night. It was an orderly progress from stages 1, 2, 3, 4, 2, REM, 2, etc. The other group consisted of the restless four subjects who tended to awaken during sleep and often drifted upward from stage 2 sleep into stage 1 or awakening (Hammack et al., 1964). Although this study was not undertaken in order to distinguish between good and poor sleepers, it certainly told of a perceptible difference between volunteers who came to the laboratory to be subjects in sleep experiments.

In our present tentative picture of a normal night's sleep there are many variations, variations that appear on other measures than the EEG. In almost every human study, scientists have spoken about the range within which subjects show the same responses. Not all subjects show exactly the same pattern on any measure, and some of these variations may help to characterize sound and restless sleep. The density of eye movements, perhaps reflecting a degree of brain stem excitation, varies in different dream periods and seems unusually high in some psychotic patients, unusually low in others. These many factors may be the first hints to tell what are the differences between good sleep and poor sleep.

The first investigation of the overall difference between good and poor sleep was performed a year ago with two matched groups of poor and good sleepers. Dr. Lawrence J. Monroe, working as a graduate student in the sleep laboratory of the University of Chicago, has shown that people who complain about their sleep really differ from those who admit they sleep well. These differences are not merely imaginings.

The volunteers for this study were attracted to the laboratory by a local advertisement and were chosen by answers to questionnaires. All were men between 20 and 40, and 16 were selected from each group, chosen so that there were no subjects with acute disorders that would disturb sleep, nor extreme insomniacs. The volunteers were matched so that each poor sleeper had an approximate counterpart among the good sleepers in age, education, and occupation. The groups did not differ notably in athletic inclinations. Each group contained students, laborers, professionals, physically active people, and inactive people. All of the participants had to meet some minimum health standards, and in obvious characteristics the outsider would have said that the two groups were very similar.

Each subject filled out the long health questionnaire, the Cornell Medical Index, and the Minnesota Multiphasic Personality Index, a test calculated to bring out dominant psychological traits and attitudes. In other respects, the laboratory procedure was straightforward and no more taxing than innumerable other studies. Each person spent a night adjusting to sleeping in the laboratory with recording devices on his body. The next night a variety of recordings were taken while he slept. Even at this stage in the procedure, the experimenters noticed that some subjects were unusually sensitive to the recording electrodes and thermistors.

Ordinarily, the process of being dressed in electrodes before retiring is relaxing, even soporific. Subjects become quite drowsy. During this study, however, some subjects gave unusual reactions, loudly complaining, while other scarcely reacted. The oversensitive subjects were poor sleepers. These people also complained of discomfort in the laboratory bedrooms, although each participant did sleep through an entire night while recordings were made of brain waves, body motions, heart rate, skin resistance, rectal temperature, skin potential, and finger pulse volume.

Physiological Differences

The data was averaged for each group, permitting the investigator to compare the main trends, and the groups differed sharply. Poor sleepers did sleep less. They took twice as long on the average to fall asleep, requiring 15 minutes, whereas the good sleepers took an average of 7 minutes. Yet more interesting was the fact that the poor sleepers estimated that it took them 59 minutes to fall asleep while the good sleepers were more accurate in describing their own behavior. The poor sleepers awakened almost twice as frequently during the night and made many more movements of the body, shifts in position. The longest anybody could have slept would have been 7 hours. The good sleepers averaged 6½ hours, the poor sleepers 5¾ hours. Such differences are often mentioned in conversation about sleep and they are now documented in this initial study.

Pronounced physiological differences are also associated with the restlessness and difficulty of the poor sleeper in falling asleep. Higher body temperature and faster pulse suggested that poor sleepers be physiologically closer to a waking state than the good sleeper must. The pulse becomes somewhat slower during sleep, ordinarily. Before falling asleep the average heart rate of the poor sleepers was 66.9 beats a minute. This dropped to 60.5 during sleep. The good sleepers showed a lower pulse rate to start with. The average rate before sleep was 60.7, and this had dropped to 56.6 during sleep. This is a considerable difference between the two groups.

Body temperature differed similarly, although the numerical difference may seem minimal on first glance. Poor sleepers had an average temperature of 98 degrees before sleep, dropping to 97.6. The good sleepers had an average temperature of 97.7 before sleep, which dropped to an average of 97.2.

A difference between the two groups of only 0.4 of a degree may look insignificant, but the entire sleep temperature range of the healthy adult is only a degree and four-tenths. So, within this range, a group difference of four-tenths of a degree is sizable.

A relationship between dream activity and body temperature has been postulated primarily because the longest dream periods occur at the nadir of our temperature cycle. This study again suggested some relationship between dreaming and temperature. The poor sleepers spent less time in REM dreaming than did the good sleepers. Good sleepers, as a group, averaged about 24 percent of their sleeping time in the REM state. The poor sleepers, as a group, averaged only 16.9 percent. This enormous difference in proportion of dreaming is not the whole story, however, because it is based on group averages. The range within the poor sleeping group was very great, yet 12 out of 16 were dreaming considerably less than the good sleepers.

Whether or not chronic dream reduction had something to do with the psychological differences between the poor sleepers and the good sleepers is a moot question. That there were pronounced differences is undeniable. In the light of some of the dream-deprivation studies of the past, it is interesting to note that a few of the poor sleepers had previously undergone psychiatric therapy. These people actually showed more dream time than the others—23 percent. Others who had never had therapy spent as little as 13 percent of their sleep in the dream state. This may have had something to do with the fact that the poor sleepers awakened about twice as often during the night, perhaps interrupting or preventing REM sleep and suggesting a higher state of arousal during sleep.

The EEG patterns of the two groups differed in the apportionment of sleep phases throughout the night. Both groups spent some of the first half of the night in stage 4, but they distributed it differently. The poor sleepers "used up" almost all of their stage 4 during the first part of the night, whereas the good sleepers had about 72 percent of their slow-wave sleep in the first half and distributed the rest over the second half of the night.

Toward the end of the night, the body temperatures of the poor sleepers were still declining, whereas the good sleepers were showing a rise in temperature about an hour and a half before they woke up. These were some of the major physiological differences, and while they were unexpectedly striking, the questionnaire pointed up even more striking psychological differences.

Psychological Differences

Although the Cornell Medical Index is often used as a quick assay of health, it is also used to gain information about psychosomatic complaints. It is a long questionnaire, and some of its questions are addressed to objective complaints: Do you need glasses to read? Others ask about more diffuse symptoms, dizziness, headaches, nausea. Included in the list are questions about subjective adjustment: "Do you feel alone and sad at a party? Do people usually understand you?" The so-called average and well adjusted person will answer "Yes" to only about five or six of these questions. The good sleepers averaged about 6.5 affirmative answers. On the other hand, the poor sleepers averaged about 23.9 affirmative answers, suggesting that they suffer more psychosomatic ailments and experiences of maladjustment than the good sleepers. Discernible differences also appeared when the experimenters scored the Minnesota Multiphasic Personality Inventory; on this the poor sleepers seemed more hypochondriacal, introverted, anxious, and neurotic than did the good sleepers.

Even this initial material strongly suggests that the differences in sleep quality are not merely differences in sleep. Poor sleepers seem distinctive in pervasive ways. Questionnaire responses suggest they have more neurotic and psychosomatic tendencies. As a group they were more restless in sleep, fell asleep more slowly, indicated higher autonomic activity in heart rate, pulse volume, and body temperature, and distributed the EEG phases of sleep differently across the night. We do not know what makes a person become a good or poor sleeper, nor the exact meaning of the physiological concomitants. But these differences appear to be thoroughgoing, reflected in attitudes, sensitivity to the laboratory and the equipment in which they slept, not merely restricted to nighttime sleep.

Sleep Quality and Constitution

The old family doctor used to aver that good sleep was the source of well-being and hale attitudes, an intuition that has been repeated for centuries without offending common sense. But there is no way of ordering a person to sleep well. Perhaps by voluntary behaviors individuals can improve their sleep. We do not know to what extent. This study raises the ugly suspicion that there may be a predisposition to sleep well or poorly, for the physiological differences reflected in sleep may, in turn, be influencing behavior. Could these physiological patterns hold clues to physical complements of neuroses? Is there something about the poor sleeper that makes him vulnerable, and overreactive to his environment? Or is lack of rest the key to his other troubles?

Disturbed sleep can be part of a vicious circle involving emotional and behavioral deterioration. Sleep loss, in itself, induces a variety of curious symptoms, and in extreme, is attended by almost psychotic symptoms. It is associated with an alteration of the body's energy metabolism. A relatively short period of sleep loss is accompanied by the production of an indole associated with stress, a chemical of the LSD or serotonin family. Commonly, the physician sees sleep disturbances during a prelude to mental breakdown, during depression, before acute psychotic episodes. The loss of a single portion of the EEG distribution has an aftermath. After REM deprivation, whether or not individuals have shown behavioral effects, they make up for lost REM time. Similarly, when deprived only of stage 4, people make up that stage of sleep by spending a compensatory proportion of sleep in stage 4. Perhaps some regular quota and distribution of the EEG phases is necessary to each individual. In severely depressed patients and psychotics during acute episodes, there are anomalous patterns within the dream period—rapid transitions between waking and dreaming, unusually high percentages of dreaming sleep (Hawkins, 1965; Hartman et al., 1964). The numerous studies of mentally ill persons, of epileptics, narcoleptics, enuretics and others all suggest a link between anomalous sleep patterns and disordered behavior. This does not say whether the mild disturbance, the neurotic signs of the poor sleeper would be alleviated by better sleep. What we have seen in these researches is that sleep is an orderly cycle involving bodily changes and altered states of consciousness, a unity of psychological and physiological transformations that is not separable from waking health and behavior. The process resembles the turning of a wheel on which it is difficult to assign a point where the motion began, but which can be braked. Therapy may be applicable at several levels, and it is possible that the poor sleeper might benefit from a drug or conditioning that improves his sleep.

Differences between the good and poor sleeper may reflect their separation from each other along a continuum, a wide range of human sleep patterns. They may be related to individual differences spotted in many other studies. Some people, for instance, reacted more than others to sleep deprivation, or dream deprivation. People's drug responses differ, and infinitesimal dose adjustments had to be made for each individual before LSD in microdosages would leave their mark on dreaming. The ration of alcohol that put one cat to sleep left another curious and lively. Individual differences have been expressed in diverse ways. Volunteers in sleep studies have differed in their ability to press switches during sleep, follow instructions, in their amenability to hypnotic suggestion during sleep, and in their ability to recall dreams. Within dream-recall studies we may be seeing two extremes of a continuum, for one person appears to sleep so deeply that his dream has vanished by the time he awakens, while another claims he does not dream, apparently confusing dream with waking, and dreaming in such a light stage of sleep that he can hear the air conditioner and other noises in the room. Many of these differences may be constitutional, the counterparts of pervasive genetic endowments that show up in personality and behavior as well as in body build, blood type, hair color, and on other physiological measures. The influence of inherited factors is enormously difficult to determine with human beings, and consequently has not been explored intensively in relation to sleep patterns. The difficulty of ascertaining constitutional factors may explain why they are so often omitted from behavioral considerations in human studies.

One of the trends shown by poor sleepers, however, may provide a means of exploring predispositions without going back into family traits and impossible genetic skeins. The poor sleeper seems to be in a somewhat heightened physiological state, before and during sleep. Is this roughly analogous to a motor that races when it should be idling? Is the poor sleeper tuned to higher arousal, hyperreactivity? Is his metabolic and neural baseline just slightly different than that of the good sleeper? Could the higher heart rate, temperature, and the numerous awakenings mean that he is overproducing neurochemicals that stimulate the arousal system, or that he underproduces chemicals that stimulate the hypnogenic inhibiting system? There are many alternative metabolic and neural adjustments that might explain this physiological difference. A braking chemical that prevents overactivity in certain cells, may be deficient. Although this is climbing into the realm of pure speculation, we are now able to ask questions that could not have been asked sensibly even a few years ago. Indeed, recent progress has been so rapid that the answers may not be far distant.

We have mapped hypnogenic and arousal pathways within the brain, triggered by chemicals that may also turn out to mediate the influences of hormones, stress products, and other substances. The hypnogenic and arousal areas are connected with subcortical regions regulating autonomic functions such as heart rate and temperature, instinctive drive responses, pleasure, or pain. The varied basic studies from which these findings emanate, may begin to explain the neural and chemical origins of the patterns of the poor sleeper. At the same time that they give a predictive and controllable understanding of the high heart rate, arousability, of the poor sleeper, they also may be explaining why he suffers psychosomatic complaints and neurosis.

By defining precisely some of the physiological

characteristics and psychological concomitants of good and poor sleep we may provide the doctor with a new diagnostic inventory. Sleep, and resistance to sleep loss, as others have suggested, may indicate how well a person can perform under stress. But by pursuing these differences between good and poor sleepers to their neural origins, we may begin to answer questions about individual differences that have long eluded our grasp. Are many neuroses the behavioral concomitants of hyperreactivity? What causes a person to be oversensitive to his environment, to pain, and to situations that leave others unscathed? Are there also people at the other end of the scale, who underreact, on whom the environment and its social teachings leave too little impression—sociopaths and psychopaths? If these tendencies are rooted in mechanisms whose signs we see in sleep, could we detect them in early childhood? Although the links between predispositions in personality and patterns of sleep may only be conjectured at this time, the clues from observed sleep patterns are clues for internal exploration. We may at least be gaining a key to pervasive patterns underlying the development of behavior, and insight into the physiological differences that may render one person vulnerable to an environment, to a family, where others are not marred. Such explorations may help to solve some of the perplexing riddles that confront investigators of many abnormal behaviors—among them the neurotic or the juvenile delinquent whose behavior differs greatly from that of his siblings.

Summary

During the last decade, scientists of many disciplines, using different instruments and inspired by different interests, have converged onto the study of sleep only to discover that they were exploring related events, fundamental processes involved in mood, behavior, memory, health and illness, sanity and madness. The contagious excitement generated by these researches has not stemmed from the many isolated and useful discoveries so much as from their convergence toward central mechanisms in the nervous system. The sleeping brains of monkeys and chimpanzees have clarified the nature of epilepsy, and the sleeping rabbit pointed to links between mood and fertility. Physiological transformations in people and sleeping animals have suggested the instinctual basis of dreams. Like the spokes of a wheel leading to the hub, seemingly unrelated studies of muscles, finger pulse volume, attention, drugs, dream and sleep loss, have shown links and have illuminated some of our puzzling sleep disorders and symptoms of mental illness. The confluence of these fragments has generated theories about the way the nervous system functions during sleep and waking, and this may explain the proliferation of sleep studies, significant even in the last year. Communication among the world-scattered scientists of sleep may explain the astonishing rate of discovery.

Less than 10 years ago, as scientists began moving across the borders of what we used to call unconsciousness, they began demonstrating that sleep was not an unconscious suspension from life, devoid of complex behavior and only tangentially related to the quality of our days. Instead, they confronted a very active brain which, in one stage of sleep, resembled waking to an amazing degree. They confronted questions about attention as well as somnolence and relaxation. They communicated with sleepers and received answering signals.

One important fulcrum was the discovery that all sleep was punctuated by intervals of rapid EEG rhythms and eye movements, and vivid dreaming, a state not unique to man, but found in mammals down to the primitive opossum. Today, the evidence suggests that the visual imagery of dreams is not man's prize but exists in the monkey and perhaps all seeing animals. Both men and animals show a need to dream, for when deprived of the REM dream state by loss of sleep, by drugs, by anxiety, or deliberate awakenings, the normal individual quickly compensates, making up the loss in subsequent sleep. Since many mental illnesses are accompanied by sleep disorders, by broken sleep, anomalous dream periods, people inevitably wondered whether and how emotional disorders related to abnormalities of the REM dreaming mechanism, perhaps coming from too little REM dreaming.

Some neurophysiologists were finding that the dream state could be brought on by directly stimulating a portion of the brain stem in animals. It was abolished if a spot were destroyed within this primitive brain area. Although the regulation of sleep and dreaming seemed to be more elaborately governed and diffused in primates and man than lower animals, this important locus in

305

the brain stem led to conjectures with many implications for the understanding of psychoses and the function of dreams. It is a very old region of the brain, one of the first to form in the developing embryo, giving evidences of its rhythms before there are signs of the cortical rhythms of sleep. Perhaps this might explain why infant animals and infant humans were found to have more of this dream-state rhythm which declined with age as the cortex matured. Perhaps, indeed, the decline of the dream state might become a measure of normal brain development in very young infants.

Further studies of the dream state suggested that it might be triggered biochemically and that loss of REM dreaming enhanced the drive oriented behaviors of animals. This in turn, suggested that a biological function of dreaming might be the development of drive mechanisms within the embryo and infant. A later function of the dream state may be the discharge of excitement in the brain's "drive centers" accompanied by a great array of psychological releases.

A most salient property of the brain, one that makes it formidable to study, is its complex interrelatedness. While many experimenters have concentrated upon the relationships between the brain stem and related regions during the dream state, other scientists have concentrated attention upon such distant brain systems as the hippocampus. Single electric stimulations to this area and other brain regions will produce the familiar brain waves of activated, or paradoxical sleep. The hippocampus has been associated with memory and emotion, has been shown to be related to the cortex and to subcortical areas, to activity in the autonomic nervous system and body muscle systems. These links may help us to learn how the contents of the inner dream experience are produced and how they are related to the physiological events seen during the REM dream state. They may also suggest some links between the state of anxiety in which an individual may be less than usually sensitive to his surroundings and the brain mechanisms producing REM dreaming. In both anxiety and dreaming a portion of the brain may be operating in almost a closed-circuit manner.

Theory is always bound to be partly wrong, but it has been the evolution of theories that encourages experiment, motivating discoveries that would otherwise be mere fragments, or might never be done. So in sleep research, theories have inspired the accumulation of data which are now beginning to fit together and explain some of the most baffling of sleep disorders. Sleepwalking is an example. Muscle flaccidity during sleep and other findings about the dream state did not jibe with the common idea that sleepwalking occurred in the REM dream state. Bedwetting and somnambulism, indeed, both occurred during other stages of sleep. Inferences from many studies of the brains of sleeping animals and people may explain how the somnambulist shambles around furniture, eyes open, yet giving no expression of seeing. During slow-wave sleep, sensory impulses flood into the brain, but the integrative regions that create perception and awareness function in an altered, delayed manner.

A new picture of narcolepsy has emerged. The attack is one of normal sleep in an abrupt drop from waking into the REM dream state, with a sudden loss of muscle tone. A seizure locus in the amygdala has been postulated and also dream loss. The amphetamines narcoleptics take in order to stay awake have been found to have a REM-reducing effect. Although the exact brain mechanism has not yet been deciphered, new diagnostic procedures and therapy have been developed out of the studies so far.

The practical consequence of sleep research extend, into every realm of living and certainly into our use of drugs. Alcohol, barbiturates, and many tranquilizers depress REM dreaming, for instance, although they differ in their impact. The effect upon neural mechanisms of dreaming may also explain hangovers, and drug psychoses. Barbiturates do more than reduce REM dream time, they interfere with integrative processes in the brain, which in turn, may be participating in maintaining body functions. It has been thought that some psychotics, or narcoleptics, or other individuals suffering from dream loss might benefit from increased dreaming. Current explorations of LSD and gamma-hydroxybutyrate suggest that a drug therapy to increase dreaming may be possible. As a result of sleep studies our use of tranquilizers, sedatives, and antidepressants, may be far less haphazard, for we are beginning to determine how they act upon the brain, why individuals react differently to the same drug, or to a particular concentration.

We are just beginning to explore the chemistry

of sleep, to see how natural body substances such as sex hormones influence sleep. Here may be the roots of many abnormalities, for slight increases in steroid hormones that produce sleep, can mean anesthesia, or convulsion. Anatomical mapping of the sleep circuit and arousal centers in the brain has employed two neurochemicals which may be the basic transmitters, the crucial chemicals that mediate sleep and arousal. Insufficient supply of the hypnogenic transmitter may cause the insomnia of the elderly, who awaken too early. Oversupply of an arousal mediator may play a role in the inability to fall asleep. Within the metabolism of the sleeping brain we may expect to find the clues to many pervasive disorders; and perhaps also pervasive personal tendencies. Do some people tend to inhibition and others to arousal? Under the horrendous conditions of battle that agitate most people, some soldiers are known to have fallen asleep in the trenches. There are many instances in which a situation fraught with emotion has caused a soporific reaction within one person, a restless reaction in another.

Very pervasive individual differences have been noted throughout sleep researches, expressed in behavior and attitude and in physiological patterns. Are these related? Are we on the way toward looking at a person's polygraph record during sleep and predicting how well he will tolerate stress, hunger, sleep loss, pain, dream deprivation? Could we learn from this sleep record about his ability to remember dreams, to perform tasks during sleep, his response to certain drugs? Could we predict from these physiological indices his propensity toward psychosomatic ailments, and the intimations of his personality that he will leave on psychological questionnaires? Does the heightened physiological state of a poor sleeper indicate a high setting within the brain's system of arousal—leading him to overreact to the environment? If so, could we detect incipient neurosis early in life? As the findings from diverse sleep studies are juxtaposed, they begin to suggest internal links, and raise innumerable questions of monumental importance to medicine and psychiatry.

These questions are beginning to be clarified by studies that may seem remote, but the scientist observing human behavior is like an astronomer with an optical telescope, recording what can be seen with the eye, while unseen and invisible radiations from that same place must be interpreted through radio antennas.

New instruments and techniques of analyzing data have become increasingly important in brain study, where most of our questions lead. Using tiny electrodes, deeply implanted in the brains of animals, researchers have begun to read what is happening in the brain during the different phases of sleep.

The discharge patterns of single brain cells, as well as groups of cells, are yielding clues about neural organization during dreaming, about the nature of hallucination, and seizure. The brain's responses to signals has enabled us to track the neural mechanisms by which a mother learns to awaken to her child's whimper, yet sleep through traffic. From studies of brain responses, averaged and analyzed by computer, we have inferred a fundamental distinction between dreaming and other deep sleep. During REM dreaming, the sensory impulses are screened out, to an extent that resembles the censorship of waking in moments of attention. Thus, the dream state appears to be a period of intense inward concentration, in which brain activity bears some resemblances to waking.

Encephalographers cannot distinguish, by eye, the many shifts of attention and subtle transformations that occur throughout waking and sleep, for massive information is hidden in the EEG. Many new mathematical techniques for analyzing the EEG data have been developed to eke out this information, to determine whether a few seconds of brain waves resemble each other in frequency distribution or power. The computer has become an essential instrument to perform the manipulations, or calculations of most sophisticated brain research, and indeed for any refined reading of the EEG. This is, of course, at the very heart of the matter. The EEG is a staple instrument for gauging the behavior of the mind, and the further refinement of EEG analyses may make it a diagnostic tool with which we may be able to discriminate between the patterns of the normal person, the neurotic and the schizophrenic. Indeed, by tracing the patterns of attention and other states of consciousness we may be able to distinguish between the many kinds of psychoses we now call schizophrenia. Mental disorders, as they are reflected in sleep patterns, may be tracked to their brain origins more precisely as these new methods come to wider use.

Neural changes and brain processes that are not

perceptible on the EEG, have been tracked by a new tool that measures changes in the electrical resistance of neural tissue. Recent studies illuminating the action of the sleeping brain have shown that the single nerve cell transmits messages in a rhythmic code composed of discharges and spaces. Impedance measurements of resistance changes which may occur in nonneural glial cells may tell how the excitability of the nerve cell is modulated by surrounding influences. Thus we may begin to find out how patterns of electric waves occur in various parts of the brain, in seizure activity like epilepsy, and the widespread changes we know as sleep.

The equipment, the mathematical analyses, and the intricate techniques of these basic investigations are expensive. The conclusions may seem incomprehensible on the surface, and distant from immediate problems of mental health. No serious scientist, probing a biological mechanism for its internal laws, would want to promise particular applications, yet the unforeseen yield of these unapproachable basic researches are what we count upon in the long run. If sleep research has produced rich and practical insights into the working of the mind, its productivity must be credited to a symbiosis and communication among the participants. Clinicians report a bizarre brain wave pattern in the brain of an epileptic patient in sleep, and studies of the chimpanzee indicate that this is a normal pattern although never observed before. Psychologists discover rapid eye movements during dreaming, and neurophysiologists trace excitement within a brain stem area through linked regions of the visual system. Curious sleep and dream patterns are observed in some psychotics, and untoward reactions to certain sedatives, and brain researches begin to explain that schizophrenia shows an impact upon attention mechanisms, upon which tranquilizers and barbiturates act differently.

As the EEG analyses become ever more refined and activities deep within the brain are further correlated with the ripples they create at the surface, the nightlong record of sleep may become one of our most useful diagnostic tools. It may tell us about the integrity of an infant's nervous system long before there is any behavior to test. It may warn us of incipient mental breakdown, allow us to prevent fatal coronaries in sleep, reveal whether drugs are beneficial or harmful. It may discriminate between people who can resist stress, and those who may be vulnerable, predict lifelong tendencies, proclivities for psychosomatic ailment and neurosis. It should not be discouraging that these are phrased as future possibilities rather than present certainties, for this area of study has scarcely had time to begin. Knowledge of our sleep patterns, our daily temperature rhythms, the impact of age and habit upon our response to sleep loss, our transitions from waking to sleep and from sleep to wakefulness should become useful to each individual as it is useful to know that one is sick when one has fever, or should not drive after drinking.

One of the very great contributions of sleep research could be the enrichment of human consciousness and enlargement of human capacities. The EEG has been used as an educational instrument

313

to teach people to recognize and control a state of consciousness they had not been aware of. Volunteers in the laboratory have learned to decrease blood pressure. The yogi's extraordinary bodily controls and voluntary immunity to pain come from roundabout disciplines. We, too, may begin to acquire such disciplines by more systematic means. If emotional states and autonomic functions can be modified by the individual, psychotherapy and the treatment of psychosomatic illness may substitute training for drugs. As we learn the determinants of sleep we may also acquire the knack of some unusual people, who induce sleep by deciding to sleep and who seem to awaken themselves by mental clocks, perhaps in a phase of sleep near arousal.

Sleep researches are beginning to offer tools of self-knowledge. People may begin to sense their cycles of alertness and drowsiness, and take advantage of the natural timing of their bodies, and minds. Attention, that subtle state whose neural components have begun to be pursued, may also become a faculty that we deliberately enhance in the young, for the control of attention is often a deciding factor in the productivity of a life. The concentration that might multiply and extend the abilities of more people, also shows its rhythms from the brain, perhaps making its first appearance in the young in the dream state. As research begins to reveal the correlates of these states it may be offering us methods of becoming acquainted with the feel of our own minds, an important step in using them.

Hardly foreseen 10 years ago, the study of sleep has extended its benefits into medicine, pharmacology, psychiatry, into the scheduling of work and rest, and into the education of the individual acquainting him with himself and the uses of his remarkable brain.

References

ACKNER, B., and PAMPIGLIONE, G. Some relationships between peripheral vasomotor and EEG changes. *J. Neurol. Neurosurg. Psychiat.*, 1957, 20 : 58–64.

ADEY, W. R. Computer applications of the frontiers of biomedical research. Proceedings of the Fall Joint Computer Conference, 1963.

ADEY, W. R., BELL, F., and DENNIS, B. J. Effects of LSD–25, psilocybin, and psilocin on temporal lobe EEG patterns and learned behavior in the cat. *Neurology*, 1962, 12.

ADEY, W. R., KADO, R. T., DIDIO, J., and SCHINDLER, W. J. Impedance changes in cerebral tissue accompanying a learned discriminative performance in the cat. *Exp. Neurol.*, 1963, 7.

ADEY, W. R., KADO, R. T., and RHODES, J. M. Sleep : cortical and subcortical recordings in the chimpanzee. *Science*, 1963, 141 : 932–933.

ADEY, W. R., and WALTER, D. O. Application of phase detection and averaging techniques in computer analysis of EEG records in the cat. *Exp. Neurol.*, 1963, 7.

AGNEW, H., WEBB, W. B., and WILLIAMS, R. L. The effect of stage 4 sleep deprivation. *EEG Clin. Neurophysiol.*, 1964, 17 : 68–70.

AKERT, K., ed. *Progress in Brain Research—Sleep Mechanisms*, Vol. 18. C. Bally, F. Hoffman-La Roche & Co., Basle, Switzerland, 1965, and American Elsevier, New York.

AKERT, K., KOELLA, P., and HESS, R., Jr. Sleep produced by electrical stimulation of the thalamus. *Amer. J. Physiol.*, 1952, 168 : 260–267.

ALLISON, T. Correlation of evoked response amplitude with REM during "rapid" sleep. APSS, Palo Alto, March 1964.

ALLISON, T. Cortical and subcortical evoked responses to central stimuli during wakefulness and sleep. *EEG Clin. Neurophysiol.*, 1965, 18: 131–139.

ALLUISI, E. A., CHILES, W. D., HALL, T. J., and HAWKES, G. R. Human group performance during confinement. Aero-space Medical Research Laboratories TDR 63–87.

AMADEO, M., and GOMEZ, E. Eye movements and dreaming in subjects with life-long blindness. APSS, 1964, Palo Alto.

ANDREEV, B. V. Sleep therapy in the neuroses. *Internatl. Behav. Sci. Series*, 1960.

ANLIKER, J. Variations in alpha voltage of the EEG and time perception. *Science*, 1963, 140: 1307–1309.

ANTROBUS, J. S., ANTROBUS, JUDITH S., and SINGER, J. L. Eye movements accompanying daydreaming, visual imagery, and thought suppression. *J. Abnorm. Soc. Psychol.*, 1964, 69: 244–252.

ANTROBUS, JUDITH S. Patterns of dreaming and dream recall. Unpublished doctoral dissertation, Columbia University, 1962.

ANTROBUS, JUDITH. Discrimination of EEG sleep stages I–REM vs. II. APSS, 1965, Washington, D.C.

ANTROBUS, JUDITH S., ANTROBUS, J. S., and FISHER, C. Discriminative responses to dreaming and nondreaming during different stages of sleep. Symposium, Research on dreams: Clinical and theoretical implications, Postgraduate Center for Mental Health, New York, March 1964.

ANTROBUS, JUDITH S., DEMENT, W. C., and FISHER, C. Patterns of dreaming and dream recall: EEG study. *J. Abnorm. Soc. Psychol.*, in press.

ARDUINI, A., and HIRAO, T. On the mechanism of the sleep pattern elicited by acute visual deafferentation. *Arch. Ital. Biol.*, 1959, 97: 140.

ARDUINI, A., and HIRAO, T. EEG synchronization elicited by light on the midpontine pretrigeminal. *Arch. Ital. Biol.*, 1960, 98 : 275.

ARDUINI, A., and PINNEO, L. R. Properties of the retina in response to steady illumination. *Arch. Ital. Biol.*, 1962, 100 : 425–448.

ARDUINI, A., and PINNEO, L. R. The tonic activity of the lateral geniculate nucleus in dark and light adaptation. *Arch. Ital. Biol.*, 1963, 101 : 493–507.

ARDUINI, A., and PINNEO, L. R. The effects of flicker and steady illumination on the activity of the cat visual system. *Arch. Ital. Biol.*, 1963, 101,, 508–529.

ARMSTRONG, R. H., BURNAP, D., JACOBSON, A., KALES, A., WARD, S., and GOLDEN, J. Gastric secretions during sleep and dreaming. APSS, 1965, Washington, D.C.

ASERINSKY, E., and KLEITMAN, N. Regularly occurring periods of eye motility and concomitant phenomena during sleep. *Science*, 1953, 118 : 273–274.

ASERINSKY, E., and KLEITMAN, N. Two types of ocular motility occurring in sleep. *J. Appl. Physiol.*, 1955, 8 : 1–10.

ASERINSKY, E., and KLEITMAN, N. A motility cycle in sleeping infants as manifested by ocular and gross bodily activity. *J. Appl. Physiol.*, 1955, 8 : 11–18.

AX, A., and LUBY, E. D. Autonomic responses to sleep deprivation. *A.M.A. Arch. Gen. Psychiat.*, 1961, 4 : 55–59.

BAILEY, S., BUCCI, L., GOSLINE, E., and KLINE, N.S., et al. Comparison of iproniazid with other amine oxidase inhibitors, including W–1544, JB–516, RO4–1018, and RO5–0700. *Ann. N.Y. Acad. Sci.*, 1959, 80 : 652–667.

BALDRIDGE, B. J., WHITMAN, R. M., and KRAMER, M. A comparison of variability of some physiological functions during dreaming while telling the dream and during dream playback. APSS, 1962, Chicago.

BALDRIDGE, B., WHITMAN, R., KRAMER, R., ORNSTEIN, P., and LANSKY, L. The effect of external physical stimuli on dream content. APSS, 1965, Washington, D.C.

BARNES, C. D., and MEYERS, F. H. Eserine and ampheta-mine; interactive effects on sleeping time in mice. *Science*, 1964, 144: 1221–1222.

BATINI, C., MORUZZI, G., PALESTINI, M., ROSSI, G. F., and ZANCHETTI, A. Effects of complete pontine transections on the sleep-wakefulness rhythm: the midpontine pre-trigeminal preparation. *Arch. Ital. Biol.*, 1959, 97: 1–12.

BAUST, W., BERLUCCHI, G., and MORUZZI, G. Changes in the auditory input in wakefulness and during the syn-chronized and desynchronized stages of sleep. *Arch. Ital. Biol.*, 1964, 102: 657–674.

BEH, H. C., and BARRATT, P. E. H. Discrimination and conditioning during sleep as indicated by the electro-encephalogram. *Science*, 1965, 147: 1470–1471.

BELL, C., SIERRA, G., BUENDIA, N., and SEGUNDO, J. P. Sensory properties of units in mesencephalic reticular formation. *J. Neurophysiol.*, 1964, 27: 961–987.

BERGER, R. J. Tonus of laryngeal muscles during sleep and dreaming. *Science*, 1961, 134: 840.

BERGER, R. J. Experimental modification of dream con-tent by meaningful verbal stimuli. *Brit. J. Psychiat.*, 1963, 109: 722–740.

BERGER, R., and MEIER, G. Deprivation of patterned vision and the eye movements of sleep. APSS, 1965, Washing-ton, D.C.

BERGER, R. J., OLLEY, P., and OSWALD, I. The EEG, eye-movements and dreams of the blind. *Quart. J. Exp. Psychol.*, 1962, 14: 183–186.

BERGER, R. J., and OSWALD, I. Effects of sleep variation on behavior, subsequent sleep, and dreaming. *J. Ment. Sci.*, 1962, 108: 457–465.

BERGER, R. J., and OSWALD, I. Eye movements during active and passive dreams. *Science*, 1962, 137: 601.

BERLUCCHI, G. Callosal activity during sleep and wake-fulness. APSS, 1965, Washington, D.C.

BERLUCCHI, G., MAFFEI, L., MORUZZI, G., and STRATA, P. EEG and behavioral effects elicited by cooling of medulla and pons. *Arch. Ital. Biol.*, 1964, 102: 372–392.

BERLUCCHI, G., MORUZZI, G., SALVI, G., and STRATA, P. Pupil behavior and ocular movements during synchronized and desynchronized sleep. *Arch. Ital. Biol.*, 1964, 102: 230–244.

BERLUCCHI, G., and STRATA, P. Palpebral asymmetry in the dark adapted owl (Atheme Noctua) following unilateral irreversible visual deafferentation. *Arch. Ital. Biol.*, 1962, 100: 248–258.

BESSMAN, S. P., and SKOLNIK, SANDRA J. Gamma Hydroxybutryate and Gamma Butyrolactone concentration in rat tissues during anesthesia. *Science*, 1964, 143: 1045.

BIRCHFIELD, R. I., SIEKER, H. O., and HEYMAN, A. Alterations in blood gases during natural sleep and narcolepsy. A correlation with the EEG stages of sleep. *Neurol.*, 1958, 8: 107–112.

BIZZI, E. Discharge patterns of lateral geniculate neurons during paradoxical sleep. APSS, 1965, Washington, D.C.

BIZZI, E., and BROOKS, D. C. Pontine reticular formation: Relation to lateral geniculate nucleus during deep sleep. *Science*, 1963, 141: 270–272.

BIZZI, E., POMPEIANO, O., and SOMOGYI, I. Vestibular nuclei; activity of single neurons during natural sleep and wakefulness. *Science*, 1964, 145: 414–415.

BOLCERT, EDWIN. The effects of thirst and a related auditory stimulation on dream reports. APSS, 1965, Washington, D.C.

BONVALLET, M., and DELL, P. Contrôle bulbaire du système réticulaire activateur. *Neurophysiologie des Etats de Sommeil*, Editions du centre National de la Recherche Scientifique, Paris, 1965.

BOWLING, G., and RICHARDS, N. Diagnosis and treatment of the narcolepsy syndrome. *Cleveland Clinic Quarterly*, 1961, 28: 38–45.

BREBBIA, D. R., and ALTSHULER, K. Z. Patterns of energy exchange during sleep and dreams. APSS, 1965. Washington, D.C.

BROOKS, D. C., and BIZZI, E. Brain stem electrical activity during deep sleep. *Arch. Ital. Biol.*, 1963, 101: 648.

BROWN, BARBARA B. Effect of alcohol on brain electrical correlates of behavior, emotional responsiveness, and visual perception in cats. Scientific Advisory Council Licensed Beverage Industries, Inc., 1964.

BROWN, BARBARA B. EEG characteristics related to personality traits in cats. 1965 preprint.

BROWN, BARBARA B., CHOPRA, S., and SHRYNE, J. E. Visual recall ability and eye movements. 1964 preprint.

BROWN, BARBARA B., SHRYNE, J. E. EEG theta activities and fast activity sleep in cats related to behavior traits. *Neuropsychologia*, 1964, 311–326.

BROWN, BARBARA B., SHRYNE, J., and DELL, MARGARET. Relationship between personality-behavior characteristics and the sleep-dream cycle in cats. APSS, 1964, Palo Alto.

BUENDIA, N. SIERRA, G., GOODE, M., and SEGUNDO, J. P. Conditioned and discriminatory responses in wakeful and in sleeping cats. *EEG Clin. Neurophysiol.*, Supp. 24, 1963, 199–218.

BULOW, K. Respiration and wakefulness in man. *Acta physiologica Scandinavia*, 1963, 59, supp. 209.

BURESOVA, O. BURES, J. FIFKOVA, E., VINOGRADOVA, O., and WEISS, T. Function significance of corticohippocampal connections. *Exper Neurol.*, 1962, 6 : 161.

CADILHAC, J., and PASSOUANT-FONTAINE, T. Decharges epileptiques et activite electrique de veille it de sommeil dans l'hippocampe au cours do l'ontogenese. *Editions du Centre National de la Recherche Scientifique*, 1962, 429–442.

CADILHAC, J., PASSOUANT-FONTAINE, T., and PASSOUANT, P. L'organisation des divers stades du sommeil chez le chaton de la naissance a 45 jours. *J. Physiol.*, 1962, 54 : 305–306.

CHAMACHO-EVANGELISTS, A., and REINOSO-SUAREZ, F. Activating and synchronizing centers in cat brain: EEGs after lesions. *Science*, 1964, 146 : 268–270.

CANDIA, O., FAVALE, E., GUISSANI, A., and ROSSI, G. Blood pressure during natural sleep and during sleep induced by electrical stimulation of the brain stem reticular formation. *Arch. Ital. Biol.*, 1962, 100 : 216–233.

CARLI, G., ARMENGOL, V., and ZANCHETTI, A. EEG desynchronization during deep sleep after destruction of midbrain-limbic pathways in the cat. *Science*, 1963, 140: 677-679.

CASPERS, H. On steady potential shifts during various stages of sleep. *Neurophysiologie des Etats de Sommeil*, Editions du Centre National de la Recherche Scientifique, Paris, 1965.

CHAPMAN, L. F., WALTER, R. D., ADEY, W. R., CRANDAL, O. H., RAND, R. W., BRAZIER, J. A. B., and MARKHAM, C. H. Altered electrical activity of human hippocampus and amygdala induced by LSD-25. *The Physiologist*, 1962, 5.

CHIN, JANE, KILLAM, EVA, and KILLAM. K. Alteration of evoked auditory potentials during states of consciousness. APSS, 1964, Palo Alto.

CHOPRA, S., DELL, M., and BROWN, B. Theta wave characteristics during orienting and during paradoxical sleep. APSS, 1964, Palo Alto.

CLARK, P. C., and WEBB, M. W. Electrosleep therapy in the neurotic and psychogenic disorders. 1963 preprint.

CLEMENTE, C. D., and STERMAN, M. B. Cortical recruitment and sleep patterns in acute restrained and chronic behaving cats. *EEG Clin. Neurophysiol.*, 1962, 14: 420.

CLEMENTE, C. D., and STERMAN, M. B. Cortical synchronization and sleep patterns in acute restrained and chronic behaving cats induced by basal forebrain stimulation. *EEG. Clin. Neurophysiol.*, supp. 24, 1963.

CLEMENTE, C. D., STERMAN, M. B., and WYRWICKA, W. Forebrain inhibitory mechanism: Conditioning of basal forebrain induced EEG synchronization and sleep. *Exp. Neurol.*, 1963, 7.

COBB, J., EVANS, F. J., GUSTAFSON, L. A., O'CONNELL, D. N., ORNE, M. T., and SHOR, R. E. Sleep-suggestion phenomena in trained hypnotic subjects: A preliminary report. Paper presented at APSS, 1964.

COBB, J., EVANS, F., GUSTAFSON, L., O'CONNELL, D. N., ORNE, M., and SHOR, R. Specific motor responses during sleep to sleep-administered meaningful suggestion: an exploratory investigation. *Percept. Mot. Skills*, 1965, 20: 629-636.

CORAZZA, DI R., and PARMEGGIANI, P. L. Desincronizza-
zione dei ritmi bioelettrci dell' ippocampo. *Arch. Sci.
Biol.*, 1961, 45 : 401.

CORDEAU, J. P. EEG and behavorial changes following
microinjections of acetylcholine and adrenaline in the
brain stem of cats. APSS, 1964, Palo Alto.

CORDEAU, J. P. Sensory transmission in the visual system
during various states of sleep and wakefulness. APSS,
1964, Palo Alto.

CREUTZFELDT, O. D., BELL, F. R., and ADEY, W. R. The
activity of neurons in the amygdala of the cat following
afferent stimulation. In W. Bergmann and J. P. Schade
(eds.), *Progress in brain research*. Amsterdam : Elsevier, 1963.

DALY, D. D., and YOSS, R. E. Electroencephalogram in
narcolepsy. *EEG Clin. Neurophysiol.*, 1957, 9 : 109–120.

DALY, D. D., and YOSS, R. E. A family with narcolepsy.
Proceedings of Staff Meetings of the Mayo Clinic, 1959,
34.

DECKERT, G. H. Pursuit eye movement in the absence of
a moving stimulus. *Science*, 1964, 143 : 1192–1193.

DE LA MARE, W. *Behold this Dreamer!* New York:
Knopf, 1939.

DELANGE, M., CASTAN, P., CADILHAC, J., and PASSOUANT,
P. Study of night sleep during centrencephalic and
temporal epilepsies. *EEG Clin. Neurophysiol.*, 1962,
14 : 777.

DELL, P., BONVALLET, M., and HUGELIN, A. Mechanisms
of reticular deactivation. In G. E. W. Wolstenholme
and M. O'Connor (eds.), *The Nature of Sleep*. Boston :
Little, Brown, 1960.

DELORME, F., VIMONT, P., and JOUVET, D. Etude statis-
tique du cycle vielle-sommeils chez le Chat. *C.R. Soc.
Biol.* 1964, 158 : 2128–2130.

DEMENT, W. C. Dream recall and eye movements during
sleep in schizophrenics and normals. *J. Nerv. Ment.
Dis.*, 1955, 122 : 263–269.

DEMENT, W. C. The occurrence of low voltage, fast, EEG patterns during behavioral sleep in the cat. *EEG Clin. Neurophysiol.*, 1958, 10 : 291–296.

DEMENT, W. C. The effect of dream deprivation. *Science*, 1960, 131 : 1705–1707.

DEMENT, W. C. An Essay on Dreams. In W. Edwards, H. Lindman, and L. D. Phillips (eds.) *New Directions in Psychology II*. New York : Holt, Rinehart & Winston, 1965.

DEMENT, W. C. Further studies on the function of rapid eye movement sleep. *Am. Psychiatric Assn.*, New York, 1965.

DEMENT, W. C. Studies on the function of rapid eye movement (paradoxical) sleep in human subjects. *Neurophysiologie des Etats de Sommeil*, Editions du Centre National de la Recherche Scientifique, Paris, 1965.

DEMENT, W. C. Experimental dream studies. In J. Masserman (ed.), *Science and psychoanalysis: Scientific proceedings of the Academy of Psychoanalysis*, vol. 7. In press.

DEMENT, W. C., and CHOW, K. Preliminary report on EEG activation during behavioral arousal and paradoxical sleep in the chronic "isolated hemisphere" preparation. APSS, 1964, Palo Alto.

DEMENT, W. C., GREENBERG, S., and KLEIN, R. The persistence of the REM deprivation effect. APSS, 1965, Washington, D.C.

DEMENT, W. C., and KLEITMAN, N. Cyclic variations in EEG during sleep and their relations to eye movements, body motility, and dreaming. *EEG Clin. Neurophysiol.*, 1957, 9 : 673–690.

DEMENT, W. C., and KLEITMAN, N. The relation of eye movements during sleep to dream activity : An objective method for the study of dreaming. *J. Exp. Psychol.*, 1957, 53 : 339–346.

DEMENT, W. C., RECHTSCHAFFEN, A., and GULEVITCH, G. D. A polygraphic study of the narcoleptic sleep attack. Abstract. *EEG Clin. Neurophysiol.*, 1964, 17 : 608–609.

DEMENT, W. C., and WOLPERT, E. A. Relationships in the manifest content of dreams occurring on the same night. *J. Nerv. Ment. Dis.*, 1958, 126: 568–578.

DEMENT, W. C., and WOLPERT, E. A. The relationship of eye movement, body motility, and external stimuli to dream content. *J. Exp. Psychol.*, 1958, 55: 543–553.

DETRE, T. DAVIS, J., and SPAULDING, P., et al. Sleep disturbance in mental patients. APSS, 1965, Washington, D.C.

DEWSON, J. H., DEMENT, W. C., WAGENER, T., NOBEL, K. A central-neural change coincident with REM sleep deprivation in cat. APSS, 1965, Washington, D.C.

DIAMOND, E. *The Science of Dreams.* New York: Mac-Fadden-Bartell, 1963.

DIAZ-GUERRO, R., GOTTLIEB, J. S., and KNOTT, J. R. The sleep of patients with manic-depressive psychosis, depressive type. An electro-myographic study. *Psychosom. Med.*, 1946, 8: 399–409.

DOMHOFF, G. W. A comparison of dream content in laboratory and home dream reports. APSS, 1963, New York.

DREYFUS-BRISAC, C., SAMSON, D., BLANC, C., and MONOD, N. L'electro-encephalogramme de l'enfant normal de-moins de 3 ans. *Etudes Neo-Natales*, 1958, 7: 143.

ELLIS, H. *The World of Dreams.* Boston: Houghton-Mifflin, 1911.

EMMONS, W. H., and SIMON, C. W. The nonrecall of material presented during sleep. *Amer. J. Psych.*, 1956, 69.

EVANS, F. J., GUSTAFSON, L. A., O'CONNELL, D. N. ORNE, M. T., and SHOR, R. E. Specific motor response during sleep to sleep-administered meaningful suggestion: Further explorations. Paper at APSS, 1965.

EVARTS, E. V. Effects of sleep and waking on activity of single units in the unrestrained cat. In G. E. W. Wolstenholme and M. O'Connor (eds.), *The Nature of Sleep.* Boston: Little, Brown, 1960.

EVARTS, E. V. Effects of sleep and waking on spontaneous and evoked discharge of single units in visual cortex. *Fed. Proc.*, 1960, 19: 828–837.

EVARTS, E. V. Activity of neurons in visual cortex of the cat during sleep with low voltage fast EEG activity. *J. Neurophysiol.*, 1962, 25 : 812–816.

EVARTS, E. V. Photically evoked responses in visual cortex units during sleep and waking. *J. Neurophysiol.*, 1963, 26 : 229–248.

EVARTS, E. V. Temporal patterns of discharge of pyramidal track neurons during sleep and waking in the monkey. *J. Neurophysiol.*, 1964, 27 : 152–171.

EVARTS, E. V. Temporal patterns of pyramidal tract neurones during sleep and waking in the monkey. *Neurophysiologie des Etats de Sommeil*, Editions du Centre National de la Recherche Scientifique, Paris, 1965.

EVARTS, E. V. Neuronal activity in visual and motor cortex during sleep and waking. Preprint.

EVARTS, E. V., BENTAL, E., BIHARI, B., and HUTTENLOCHER, P. Spontaneous discharge of single neurons during sleep and waking. *Science*, 1962, 135 : 726–728.

FAIR, C. M. *The Physical Foundations of the Psyche.* Wesleyan University Press, 1963.

FAURE, J. The paradoxical phase of sleep in the rabbit— its neurohormonal relationship. *EEG Clin. Neurophysiol.*, 1962, 14 : 784.

FAURE, J., and BENSCH, C. Mesencephale et "post-reaction-EEG" dans le comportement lié à la view endocrino-genitale du lapin. *Rev. Neurol.*, 1962, 106 : 197–201.

FAURE, J., BENSCH, C., and VINCENT, D. Role d'un systeme mesencephalolimbique dans la "phase paradoxale" du sommeil chez le lapin. *C.R. Soc. Bio.*, 1962, 156 : 70–73.

FAVALE, E., LOEB, C., and MANFREDI, M. Somatic evoked potentials during the different phases of sleep in cats. *EEG Clin. Neurophysiol.*, 1963, 15 : 917.

FAVALE, E., LOEB, C., ROSSI, G. F., and SACCO, G. EEG synchronization and behavioral signs of sleep following low frequency stimulation of the brain stem reticular formation. *Arch. Ital. Biol.*, 1961, 99 : 1–22.

FEINBERG, I., KORESKO, R. L., GOTTLEIB, F., and WENDER, P. H. Sleep electroencephalographic and eye-movement patterns in schizophrenic patients. *Comp. Psychiat.*, 1964, 5: 44-53.

FEINBERG, I., LANE, M. H., LASSES, N. A. Senile dementia and cerebral oxygen uptake measured on the right and left sides. *Nature*, 1960, 188: 962-964.

FELDMAN, S. Neurophysiological mechanisms modifying afferent hypothalamus-hippocampal conduction. *Exper. Neurol.*, 1962, 5: 269.

FISCHGOLD, A., and SCHWARTZ, B. A. A clinical, electroencephalographic and polygraphic study of sleep in the human adult. In G. E. W. Wolstenholme and M. O'Connor (eds.), *The Nature of Sleep*. Boston: Little, Brown, 1960, 209-236.

FISHBEIN, W., SCHAUMBERG, H., and WEITZMANN, E. D. Rapid eye movements during sleep in dark reared kittens. APSS, 1965, Washington, D.C.

FISHER, A. E. Chemical stimulation of the brain. *Scientific American*, 1964, 210: 60-68.

FISHER, C. Psychoanalytic implications of recent research on sleep and dreaming. *J. Amer. Psychoanal. Ass.*, 1965, April.

FISHER, C., and DEMENT, W. C. Studies on the psychopathology of sleep and dreams. *Amer. J. Psychiat.*, 1963, 119: 1160-1168.

FISHER, C., GROSS, J., and ZUOH, J. A cycle of penile erections synchronous with dreaming (REM) sleep. *Arch. Gen. Psychiatry*, 1965, 12: 29-45.

FISK, H., KLEIN, G. S., and BOKERT, E. Waking fantasies following interruption of two types of sleep. *Arch. Gen. Psychiat.*, In press.

FOULKES, D. Dream reports from different stages of sleep. *J. Abnorm. Soc. Psychol.*, 1962, 65: 14-25.

FOULKES, D. Theories of dream formation and recent studies of sleep consciousness. *Psychol. Bull.*, 1964, 62: 236-247.

FOULKES, D., and RECHTSCHAFFEN, A. Presleep determinants of dream content: The effects of two films. *Per. Mot. Skills*, 1964, 19: 983–1005.

FOULKES, D., and VOGEL, G. Mental activity at sleep onset. *J. Abnorm. Psychol.* In press.

FREEMAN, F. R., AGNEW, Jr., H. W., and WILLIAMS, R. L. An EEG study of the effects of meprobamate on human sleep. *Clin. Pharmacol. Ther.*, 1965, 6: 172–176.

FREUD, S. *The Interpretation of Dreams.* New York: Basic Books, 1955.

FUCHS and WU. Sleep with half-open eyes. *Amer. J. Ophthal.*, 1948, 31.

GANADA, W. The narcolepsy syndrome. *Neurol.*, 1958, 8: 487–496.

GASTAUT, H., BATINI, C., and FRESSY, J. On epileptic attacks recorded during the night sleep of epileptic children. *EEG Clin. Neurophysiol.*, 1963, 15: 142.

GASTAUT, H., and BROUGHTON, R. J. Conclusions concerning the mechanism of enuresis nocturna. *EEG Clin. Neurophysiol.*, 1964, 16: 625.

GASTAUT, H., and ROTH, B. A propos des manifestations electroencephalographiques de 140 cas de narcolepsie avec ou sans cataplexie. *Rev. Neurol.*, 1957, 97: 388–393.

GIARMAN, N. J., and ROTH, R. H. Differential estimation of gamma-butyrolactone and gamma-hydroxybutyric acid in rat blood and brain. *Science*, 1964, 145: 583–584.

GOFF, W. R., ROSNER, B. S., and ALLISON, T. Distribution of cerebral somatosensory evoked responses in normal man. *EEG Clin. Neurophysiol.*, 1962, 14: 697–713.

GOODENOUGH, D. R. Cyclical fluctuations in sleep-depth and eye-movement activity during the course of natural sleep. *Canad. Psychiat. J.*, 1963, 8: 406–408.

GOODENOUGH, D. R., LEWIS, H. B., SHAPIRO, A., JARET, L., and SLESER, I. Dream reporting following abrupt and gradual awakenings from different types of sleep. *J. Pers. and Soc. Psychol.*, 1965, 2, 170–179.

GOODENOUGH, D. R., LEWIS, H. B., SHAPIRO, A., and SLESER, I. Some factors affecting recall of dreams after laboratory awakenings. Reprint.

GOODENOUGH, D. R., SHAPIRO, A., HOLDEN, M., and STEIN-
SCHREIBER, L. A comparison of "dreamers" and "non-
dreamers": Eye movements, electroencephalograms,
and the recall of dreams. *J. Abnorm. Soc. Psychol.*,
1959, 62: 295–302.

GRANDA, A. M., and HAMMACK, J. T. Operant behavior
during sleep. *Science*, 1961, 133: 1485–1486.

GRASTYAN, ENDRE. The hippocampus and higher nervous
activity. In M. Brazier (ed.), *The Central Nervous
System and Behavior.* The Josiah Macy Foundation,
1959.

GREEN, J. D., and ARDUINI, A. A. Hippocampal electrical
activity in arousal. *J. Neurophysiol*, 1954, 17: 533.

GREEN, W. J. The effect of LSD on the sleep-dream cycle.
An exploratory study. *J. Nerv. and Ment. Dis.* In press.

GREENBERG, R. M. Cortical sensory lesions and dream and
sleep patterns. APSS, 1965, Washington, D.C.

GREENBERG, R. M., and LEIDERMAN, P. H. Perceptions, the
dream process, and memory. APSS, 1965, Palo Alto.

GREENBERG, R. M., and PEARLMAN, C. Delirium tremens
and dream deprivation. APSS, 1964, Palo Alto.

GRESHAM, S. C., AGNEW, Jr., H. W., and WILLIAMS, R. L.
"The Sleep of Depressed Patients: An EEG and Eye
Movement Study." Accepted Apr. 6, 1965. *Arch. Gen.
Psychiatry.*

GRESHAM, S. C., WEBB, W. B., and WILLIAMS, R. L. Alcohol and caffeine: effects on inferred visual dreaming.
Science, 1963, 140: 1226–1227.

GROSS, J., FELDMAN, M., and FISHER, C. Eye movements
during emergent stage 1 EEG in subjects with lifelong
blindness. APSS, 1965, Washington, D.C.

GROSS, M. M., GOODENOUGH, D., TOBIN, M., HALPERT, E.,
DOMINICK, L., PERLSTEIN, A., SIROTA, M., DiBIANCO, J.,
FULLER, RUTH, and KISHNER, I. Sleep Disturbances and
Hallucinations in the Acute Alcoholic Psychosis. APSS,
1964, Palo Alto.

GUZAAI, M., and ZANCHETTI, A. Carotid sinus and aortic
reflexes in the regulation of circulation during sleep.
Science, 1965, 148: 397–398.

GULEVITCH, G., and DEMENT, W. All-night sleep recordings
in schizophrenics in remission. APSS, 1964, Palo Alto.

HALL, C. What people dream about. *Scientific American*, 1951, 184 : 60–63.

HALL, C. S. A cognitive theory of dream symbols. *J. Gen. Psychol.*, 1953, 48 : 169–186.

HALL, C. S. A cognitive theory of dreams. *J. Gen. Psychol.* 1953, 49 : 273–282.

HALL, C. S. *The Meaning of Dreams.* New York : Dell, 1959.

HALL, C. S. Strangers in dreams : an empirical confirmation of the Oedipus complex. *J. Personality*, 1963, 31 : 336–345.

HALL, C. S. Slang and dream symbols. *Psychoanalysis and Psychoanalytic Review*, 1964. In press.

HALL, C., and DOMHOFF, B. A ubiquitous sex difference in dreams. *J. Abnor. & Soc. Psych.*, 1963, 66 : 278–280.

HALL, C., and VAN DE CASTLE, R. L. A comparison of home and monitored dreams. APSS, 1964, Palo Alto.

HALL, C., and VAN DE CASTLE, R. L. *The Content Analysis of Dreams.* Appleton-Century-Crofts, 1965.

HAMMACK, J. T. An experimental analysis of behavior during sleep. Three annual progress reports to the Defense Documentation Center—1962, 1963, and 1964.

HAMMACK, J. T., WILLIAMS, J. M., WEISBERG, P., BROOKS, PAULA, and GERARD, MARYANN. An experimental analysis of behavior during sleep. U.S. Army Medical Research and Development Command, 1964, Contract No. Da-49-193-MD-2180.

HARTMANN, E. L. Dreaming sleep and the menstrual cycle. APSS, 1965, Washington, D.C.

HARTMAN, E. L. Serotonin and dreaming sleep. APSS, 1965, Washington, D.C.

HARTMANN, E. L., VERDONE, P., and SNYDER, F. A longitudinal study of sleep and dream patterns in psychiatric patients. APSS, 1964, Palo Alto.

HAURI, P., and RECHTSCHAFFEN, A. An unsuccessful attempt to find physiological corrolates of NREM recall. APSS, 1963, New York.

HAWKINS, D. R., KNAPP, R., SCOTT, J. and THRASHER, G. Sleep studies in depressed patients. APSS, 1965, Washington, D.C.

HAWKINS, D. R., PURYEAR, H. B., WALLACE, C. D., DEAL, W. B., and THOMAS, E. S. Basal skin resistance during sleep and dreaming. *Science*, 1962, 136 : 321–322.

HAWKINS, D. R., SCOTT, J., and THRASHER, G., Sleep patterns in enuretic children. APSS, 1965.

HENRY, P., COHEN, H., STADEL, B., STULCE, J., FERGUSON, J., WAGENER, T., and DEMENT, W. CSF transfer from REM deprived cats to nondeprived recipients. APSS, 1965, Washington, D.C.

HERNANDEZ-PEON, R. Influence of attention and suggestion upon subcortical evoked electric activity in the human brain. In *EEG, Clinical Neurophysiology and Epilepsy*, Vol. III. Proceedings of the First International Congress of Neurological Sciences, Brussels, 1957. New York: Pergamon Press, 1959.

HERNANDEZ-PEON, R. Centrifugal control of sensory inflow to the brain and sensory perception. *Acta Neurol. Latinoamer.*, 1959, 5 : 279–298.

HERNANDEZ-PEON, R. Neurophysiological correlates of habituation and other manifestations of plastic inhibition. H. H. Jasper and G. D. Smirnov (eds.), *EEG Clin. Neurophysiol.*, supplement, 1960, 13 : 101–114.

HERNANDEZ-PEON, R. Olfactory bulb activity during sleep induced by stimulation of limbic structures. *Acta Neurol. Latinoamer.*, 1961, 7 : 299.

HERNANDEZ-PEON, R. Reticular mechanisms of sensory control. Massachusetts Institute Symposium on Principles of Sensory Communication. In *Sensory Communication*. New York, London: The M.I.T. Press and John Wiley & Sons, 1961.

HERNANDEZ-PEON, R. International symposium on the physiological basis of mental activity. *EEG Clin. Neurophysiol.*, 1962, 14 : 419–430.

HERNANDEZ-PEON, R. Sleep induced by localized electrical or chemical stimulation of the forebrain. *EEG Clin. Neurophysiol.*, 1962, 14 : 423–424.

HERNANDEZ-PEON, R. Atropine blockade within a cholinergic hypnogenic circuit. *Exp. Neurol.*, 1963, 8 : 20–29.

HERNANDEZ-PEON, R. Limbic cholinergic pathways involved in sleep and emotional behavior. *Exp. Neurol.*, 1963, 8 : 93–111.

331

HERNANDEZ-PEON, R. Neurophysiological mechanisms of wakefulness and sleep. XVII International Congress of Psychology, 1963, Washington, D.C.

HERNANDEZ-PEON, R. Attention, sleep, motivation and behavior. In R. Heath (ed.), *The Role of Pleasure in Behavior.* New York: Hoeber-Harper, 1964.

HERNANDEZ-PEON, R. Brain mechanisms of sleep and dreaming. Joint meeting of the Mexican Society of Neurology and Psychiatry and American Psychiatric Association, Mexico City, May 1964.

HERNANDEZ-PEON, R. A cholinergic hypnogenic limbic forebrain-hindbrain circuit. *Neurophysiologie des Etats de sommeil.* Editions du Centre National de la Recherche Scientifique, Paris, 1965.

HERNANDEZ-PEON, R. A neurophysiological model of dreams and hallucinations. *J. Nerv. Ment. Dis.* In press.

HERNANDEZ-PEON, R., and CHAVEZ-IBARRA, G. Sleep induced by electrical or chemical stimulation of the forebrain. *EEG Clin. Neurology,* supp. 24, 1962.

HERNANDEZ-PEON, R., CHAVEZ-IBARRA, G. Sleep induced by electrical or chemical stimulation of the forebrain. In R. Hernandez-Peon (ed.), *The Physiological Basis of Mental Activity. EEG Clin. Neurophysiol.,* supp. 24: 188–198, 1963.

HERNANDEZ-PEON, R., CHAVEZ-IBARRA, G., MORGANE, I. P., and TIMO-IARIA, C. Cholinergic pathways for sleep, alertness and rage in the limbic midbrain circuit. *Neurol. Latinoamer.,* 1962, 8: 93.

HESS, E. H., and POLT, J. M. Pupil size in relation to mental activity during simple problem-solving. *Science,* 1964, 140: 1190.

HEUSER, G., BUCHWALD, N. A., and WYERS, E. J. The "caudate-spindle" II: Facilitatory and inhibitory caudate-cortical pathways. *EEG Clin. Neurophysiol.,* 1961, 14: 519–524.

HOBSON, J. A. L'activite electrique phasique du cortex et du thalamus au cours du sommeil desynchronise chez le chat. *C.R. Soc. Biol.,* 1964, 158: 2131.

HOBSON, J. A. The effect of LSD on the sleep cycle of the cat. *EEG Clin. Neurophysiol.*, 1964, 17: 52–56.

HOBSON, J. A., GOLDFRANK, F., and SNYDER, F. Respiration and mental activity in sleep. *J. Psychiat. Res.* In press.

HODES, R. Ocular phenomena in the two stages of sleep in the cat. *Exp. Neurol.*, 1964, 9: 36–42.

HODES, R., and DEMENT, W. C. Abolition of electrically induced reflexes (EIR's of H reflexes) during rapid eye movement (REM) periods of sleep in normal subjects. *EEG Clin. Neurophysiol.*, 1964, 17 (Dec.).

HODES, R., and SUZUKI, J. Comparative thresholds for cortico-spinal and vestibulo-spinal movements, and for reticular formation arousal in the cat, in wakefulness, sleep, and periods of rapid eye movements. *EEG Clin. Neurophysiol.*, 1965, 18: 239–248.

HUTTENLOCHER, P. R. Evoked and spontaneous activity in single units of medial brain stem during natural sleep and waking. *J. Neurophysiol.*, 1961, 24: 451–468.

IWATA, K. and SNIDER, R. S. Cerebello-hippocampal influences on the electroencephalogram. *EEG Clin. Neurophysiol.*, 1959, 11: 439.

IZQUIERDO, I., WYRWICKA, W., SIERRA, G., and SEGUNDO, J. P. Establishment of trace reflexes during natural sleep in the cat. In Masson et Cie, *Actualities Neurophysiologiques.* In press.

JACOBSON, A., KALES, A., LEHMANN, D., and HOEDEMAKER, F. S. Muscle tonus in human subjects during sleep and dreaming. *Exp. Neurol.*, 1964, 10: 418–424.

JACOBSON, A., KALES, A., LEHMANN, D., and ZWEIZIG, J. R. Somnambulism: All night EEG studies. *Science*, 1965, 148: 975–977.

JEANNERET, P. R., and WEBB, W. B. Strength of grip on arousal from a full night's sleep. *Percept. Mot. Skills*, 1963, 17: 759–761.

JEANNEROD, M., and MOURET, J. Etude comparative des mouvements oculaires observes chez le chat au cours de da veille et du sommeil. *C.R. Soc. Biol.*, 1962, 156: 1407–1410.

JEANNEROD, M., MOURET, J., and JOUVET, M. Etude de la motricite oculaire au cours de la phase paradoxale du sommeil chez le chat. *EEG Clin. Neurophysiol.*, 1965, 18: 554–566.

JOHNSON, L., SLYE, E., and DEMENT, W. EEG and autonomic activity during and after prolonged sleep deprivaation. *Psychosomatic Med.*, 1965.

JOUVET, DANIELLE, VALATX, J. L., and JOUVET, M. Etude polygraphic de sommeil du chaton. *C.R. Soc. Biol.*, 1961, 155: 1660.

JOUVET, DANIELLE, VALATX, J. L., and JOUVET, M. Etude polygraphique du sommeil chez l'agneau. *C.R. Soc. Biol.*, 1962, 156: 1411–1414.

JOUVET, M. Telencephalic and rhombencephalic sleep in the cat. In G. E. W. Wolstenholme and M. O'Connor (eds.), *The Nature of Sleep.* Boston: Little, Brown, 1960, 188–206.

JOUVET, M. Recherches sur les mecanismes neurophysiologiques du sommeil et de l'apprentissage negatif. In J. F. Delafresnaye (ed), *Brain Mechanisms and Learning.* Oxford: Blackwell, 1961.

JOUVET, M. Ontogenetic and phylogenetic studies of sleep. APSS, 1962, Chicago.

JOUVET, M. Recherches sur les structures nerveuses et les mecanisms responsables des differentes phases du sommeil physiologique. *Arch. Ital. Biol.*, 1962, 100: 125–206.

JOUVET, M. An automatic recorder of the rhombencephalic phases of sleep in the cat: the oneirograph. *EEG Clin. Neurophysiol.*, 1963, 15: 141.

JOUVET, M. Etude du sommeil chez le chat pontique chronique. Colloque international du Centre National de la Recherche Scientifique: Aspects anatomo-fonctionnels de la physiologie du sommeil, Lyon, September, 1963.

JOUVET, M. The rhombencephalic phase of sleep. In G. Moruzzi, A. Fessard, and H. H. Jasper (eds.), *Progress in Brain Research*, vol. 1, Amsterdam: Elsevier Publishing Co., 1963.

JOUVET, M. Etude de la dualite des etats de sommeil et des mecanismes de la phase paradoxale. In *Aspects Anatomo-fonctionnels de la physiologie du sommeil*, C.N.R.S., 1965.

JOUVET, M. Paradoxical sleep—a study of its nature and mechanisms. In K. Akert, C. Bally, and J. P. Schade, (eds.), *Sleep Mechanisms*, vol. 18, Elsevier, Amsterdam, 1965.

JOUVET, M. Neurophysiology of the states of sleep. *Physiological Reviews*. In press.

JOUVET, M., CIER, A., MOUNIER, DANIELLE, and VALATX, J. Effets du 4-butyrolactone et du 4-hydroxybutyrate de sodium sur l'EEG et le comportement du chat. *C.R. Soc. Biol.*, 1961, 155 : 1313–1316.

JOUVET, M., and JOUVET, D. A study of the neurophysiological mechanisms of dreaming. *EEG Clin. Neurophysiol., supplement*, 1963, 24 : 133–156.

JOUVET, M., and JOUVET, D. Le sommeil et les reves chez l'animal. Psychiatre Animale: Bibliotheque Neuropsychiatrique de langue Francaise, 1964.

JOUVET, M., JOUVET, D., and VALATX, J. L. Etude du sommeil chez le chat pontique. Sa suppression automatique. *Comptes rendus des seances de la Societe de Biologie*, 1963, 157 : 845.

JOUVET, M., and MOUNIER, D. Effets des lesions de la formation reticulee pontique sur le sommeil du chat. *C.R. Soc. Biol.*, 1960, 154 : 2301.

JOUVET, M., and MOUNIER, D. Neurophysiological mechanisms of dreaming. *EEG Clin. Neurophysiol.*, 1962, 14 : 424.

JOUVET, M., PELLIN, B., and MOUNIER, D. Etude polygraphique des differentes phases du sommeil au cours des troubles de conscience chroniques (comas prolonges). *Revue Neurologique*, 1961, 105 : 181–186.

JOUVET, M., PELLIN, B., and MOUNIER, D. Polygraphic study of the different sleep phases during chronic disturbances of consciousness (prolonged comas). *EEG Clin. Neurophysiol.*, 1962, 14 : 138.

KAHN, E., DEMENT, W., FISHER, C., and BARMACK, J. Incidence of color in immediately recalled dreams. *Science*, 1962, 137 : 1054–1055.

KALES, A., HOEDEMAKER, F. S., and JACOBSON, A. Reportable mental activity during sleep. APSS, 1963, New York.

KALES, A., HOEDEMAKER, F. S., JACOBSON, A. and LICHTENSTEIN, E. L., Dream deprivation: an experimental reappraisal. *Nature*, 1964, 204: 1337-1338.

KAMIYA, J. Behavioral, subjective, and physiological aspects of drowsiness and sleep. In D. W. Fiske and S. R. Maddi (eds.), *Functions of Varied Experience*. Homewood: Dorsey, 1961.

KAMIYA, J. Behavioral and physiological concomitants of dreaming. APSS, 1962, Chicago.

KAMIYA, J. Conditioned discrimination of the EEG alpha rhythm in humans. Western Psychological Association, 1962.

KANEMATSU, S., and SAWYER, C. H., Effects of hypothalamic estrogen implants on pituitary LH and prolactin in rabbits. *Amer. J. Physiol.*, 1963, 205: 1073-1076.

KANEMATSU, S., and SAWYER, C. H. Effects of hypothalamic and hypophysial implants on pituitary gonadotropic cells in ovariectomized rabbits. *Endocrinology*, 1963, 73: 687-695.

KANEMATSU, S., and SAWYER, C. H. Effects of intrahypothalamic implants of reserpine on lactation and pituitary prolactin in the rabbit. *Proc. Soc. Exper. Biol. & Med.*, 1963, 113: 967-969.

KARACAN, I., GOODENOUGH, D. R., SHAPIRO, A., and WITKIN, H. A. Some psychological and physiological correlates of penile erections during sleep. APSS, 1965, Washington, D.C.

KAUFMAN, E., ROFFWARG, H., and MUZIO, J. Alterations in the sleep EEG configuration of a drug addict during addiction, withdrawal, and baseline nights. APSS, 1964, Palo Alto.

KAUFMAN, E., ROFFWARG, H., MUZIO, J. Alterations in the sleep EEG configuration during narcotic addiction, withdrawal, and post-withdrawal states. APSS, 1964, Palo Alto.

KAWAKAMI, J., and SAWYER, C. H. Induction of behavioral and electro-encephalographic changes in the rabbit by hormone administration or brain stimulation. *Endocrinology*, 1959, 65: 631-643.

KAWAKAMI, M., and SAWYER, C. H. Induction of "paradoxical" sleep by conditioned stimulation in the rabbit. *The Physiologist*, 1962, 5: 165.

KAWAMURA, H., and SAWYER, C. H. D.C. potential changes in the rabbit during slow wave sleep, paradoxical sleep, and wakefulness. *Amer. J. Physiol.*, 1964, December.

KAWAMURA, H., and SAWYER, C. H. Differential temperature changes in the rabbit brain during slow wave and paradoxical sleep. APSS, 1965, Washington, D.C.

KEEFE, W. P., YOSS, R. E., MARTENS, T. G., and DALY, D. D. Ocular manifestations of narcolepsy. *Amer. J. Ophth.* 1960, 49: 953–957.

KETY, S. S. Sleep and the energy metabolism of the brain. In G. E. W. Wolstenholme and M. O'Connor (eds.), *The Nature of Sleep*. Boston: Little, Brown, 1960, 375–381.

KHAZAN, N., and SAWYER, C. "Rebound" recovery from deprivation of paradoxical sleep in the rabbit. *Proc. Soc. Exp. Biol. Med.*, 1963, 114: 536–539.

KING, E., and McDONALD, D. G. Correlates of sleep disturbance in psychiatric patients. APSS, 1965, Washington, D.C.

KING, P., McGINTY, D., and ROBERTS, L. Recovery of function in the forebrain of the *cerveau isole* cat. APSS, 1964, Palo Alto.

KLEIN, M. *Etude polygraphique et phylogenique des etats de sommeil.* Lyon: Bosc Freres, 1963.

KLEIN, M., MICHEL, F., and JOUVET, M. Etude polygraphique des etats de sommeil chez les oiseaux. *C.R. Soc. Biol.* 1964, 158: 99–103.

KLEITMAN, N. Patterns of dreaming. *Scientiflo American*, 1960, 203: 82–88.

KLEITMAN, N. The nature of dreaming. In G. E. W. Wolstenholme and M. O'Connor, (eds.), *The Nature of Sleep*, Boston: Little, Brown, 1961, 349–374.

KLEITMAN, N. *Sleep and Wakefulness.* (Rev. ed.) Chicago: University of Chicago Press, 1963.

KLINE, N. S. Comprehensive therapy of depressions. *J. Neuropsychiat.*, 1961, supp. 1, 15–26.

KOELLA, W. P. Zum Wirkungsmechanismus von Serotonin auf das Zentralnervensystem. *Praxis*, 1962, 51: 1.

KOELLA, W. P., and CZICMAN, J. Effect of intracarotid serotonin on spinal reflexes. *Fed. Proc.*, 1961, pt. 1, 20: 305.

KOELLA, W. P. and CZICMAN, J. S. Influence of serotonin upon optic evoked potentials, EEG, and blood pressure of cat. *Am. J. Physiol.*, 1963, 204: 873.

KOELLA, W. P. and FERRY, A. Cortico-subcortical homeostasis in the cat's brain. *Science*, 1963, 142: 586–589.

KOELLA, W. P., SMYTHIES, J. R., BULL, D. M., and LEVY, C. K. Physiological fractionation of the effect of serotonin on evoked potentials. *Am. J. Physiol.* 1960, 198: 205.

KOELLA, W. P., SMYTHIES, J. R., LEVY, C. K., and CZICMAN, J. Modulatory influence on cerebral cortical optic response from the carotid sinus area. *Am. J. Physiol.* 1960, 199: 381.

KOELLA, W. P., TRUNCA, C. M., and CZICMAN, J. S. Serotonin: effect on recruiting responses of the cat. *Life Sci.*, 1965, 4: 173–181.

KORANYI, E. K., and LEHMAN, H. E. Experimental sleep deprivation in schizophrenic patients. *Arch. Gen. Psychiat.*, 1960, 2: 534–544.

KORESKO, R. L., SNYDER, F., and FEINBERG, I. "Dream time" in hallucinating and non-hallucinating schizophrenic patients. *Nature*, 1963, 199: 1118-1119.

KORNETSKY, C., MIRSKY, A. F., KESSLER, E. K., and DORF, J. E. The effects of dextro-amphetamine on behavioral deficits produced by sleep loss in humans. *J. Pharmacol. Exp. Therapeut.* 1959, 127.

KULIKOV, V. N. On the problem of hypnopedia. *Soviet Psych. & Psychiat.*, 1964, 3: 13–22.

LENA, C., and PARMEGGIANI, P. L. Hippocampal theta rhythm and activated sleep. *Helv. Physiol. Acta.*, 1964, 22: 120.

LESTER, B. K. Sleep patterns of mothers and infants. APSS, 1962, Chicago.

LESTER, B. K., and BURCH, N. R. Psychophysiological studies of sleep in schizophrenic and control populations. *Am. Psychiat. Assn.*, New York, 1965.

338

LESTER, D. A new method for the determination of the effectiveness of sleep-inducing agents in humans. *Comp. Psychiat.*, 1960, 1: 301–307.

LEVIN, M. Premature waking and post-dormital paralysis. *J. Nerv. Ment. Dis.*, 1957, 125: 140–141.

LEVITT, R. A. Sleep as a conditioned response. *Psychon. Sci.*, 1964, 1: 273–274.

LEVITT, R. A., and WEBB, W. B. Effect of aspartic acid salts on exhaustion produced by sleep deprivation. *J. Pharmaceut. Sci.*, 1964, 53: 1125–1126.

LEWIS, H. B. Individual differences among reporters and non-reporters in failure to recall dreams. APSS, 1963, New York.

LEWIS, H. B., BERTINI, M., and WITKIN, H. A. Hypnagogic reverie and subsequent dreams. APSS, 1964, Palo Alto.

LIBERSON, W. T. Problem of sleep and mental disease. *Dig. Neurol. & Psychiat.*, 13, 1945. The Institute of Living, Hartford, Conn.

LIBERSON, W. T. and LIBERSON, CATHRYN W. EEG, reaction time, eye movements, respiration and mental content during drowsiness. APSS, 1965.

LINDSLEY, D. F., WENDT, R. H., FUGETT, R., LINDSLEY, D. B., and ADEY, W. R. Diurnal activity cycles in monkeys under prolonged visual pattern deprivation. *J. Comp. Physiol. Psych.*, 1962, 55: 633–640.

LISK, R. D., KRANSWISCHER, L. R. Light: evidence for its direct effect on hypothalamic neurons. *Science*, 1964, 146: 272–273.

LISSAK, K., KARMOS, G., and GRASTYAN, E. A peculiar dream-like stage of sleep in the cat. *Act. Nerv. Sup.* 1962, 4: 347.

LOVELAND, NATHENE T. and WILLIAMS, H. L. Adding, sleep loss, and body temperature. *Percept. Mot. Skills*, 1963, 16: 923–929.

LUBIN, A., and WILLIAMS, H. L. Sleep loss, tremor, and the conceptual reticular formation. *Percept. Mot. Skills*, 1959, 9: 237–239.

LUBY, E. D., FROHMAN, C. E., GRISELL, J. L., LENZO, J. E., and GOTTLIEB, J. S. Sleep deprivation: Effects on behavior, thinking, motor performance, and biological energy transfer systems. *Psychosom. Med.*, 1960, 22: 182–192.

LUBY, E. D., GRISELL, J. L., FROHMAN, C. E., LEES, H., COHEN, B. D., and GOTTLIEB, J. S. Biochemical, psychological, and behavioral responses to sleep deprivation. *Ann. N.Y. Acad. Sci.*, 1961, 96 : 71–78.

MACLEAN, P. D. Psychosomatic disease and the "Visceral Brain." *Psychosom. Med.*, 1949, 11 : 338–353.

MACLEAN, P. D. New findings relevant to the evolution of psychosexual function of the brain. *J. Nerv. Ment. Dis.*, 1962, 135 : 289–301.

MACLEAN, P. D., DENNISTON, R. H., DUA, S. Further studies on cerebral representation of penile erection : caudal thalamus, midbrain, and pons. *J. Neurophysiol.*, 1963, 26 : 273–293.

MACLEAN, P. D., DUA, S., DENNISTON, R. H. Cerebral localization for scratching and seminal discharge. *Arch. Neurol.*, 1963, 9 : 485-497.

MACLEAN, P. D., and PLOOG, D. W. Cerebral representation of penile erection. *J. Neurophysiol.*, 1962, 25 : 29–55.

MACLEAN, P. D., PLOOG, D. W., ROBINSON, B. W. Circulatory effects of limbic stimulation, with special reference to the male genital organ. *Physiol. Rev.*, 1960, 40 : 105–112.

MACWILLIAMS, J. A. Blood pressure and heart action in sleep and dreams. *Brit. Med. J.*, 1923, 2 : 1196–1200.

MANDELL, A. Biochemical aspects of rapid eye movement sleep. *Am. Psychiat. Assn.*, New York, 1965.

MANDELL, A. J., CHAPMAN, L. F., RAND, R. W., and WALTER, R. D. Plasma corticosteroids : changes in concentration after stimulation of hippocampus and amygdala. *Science.* 1963, 139 : 1212.

MANDELL, A. J. KOLAR, E. J., and SABBAT, I. Starvation, sleep deprivation and the stress responsive indole substance. *Arch. Biol. Psychiat.* In press.

MANDELL, A. J., SLATER, G., MERSOL, I., and GEERTSMA, R. H. Stress-responsive indole substance. *Arch. Gen. Psychiat.*, 1963, 9 : 89-95.

MANDELL, M. P., MANDELL, A. J., and JACOBSON, A. Biochemical and Neurophysiological Studies of Paradoxical Sleep. *Recent Advances in Biological Psychiatry*, 7 : 115–124, J. Wortis, (ed.), Plenum, N. Y., 1965.

MANZONI, T. and PARMEGGIANI, P. L. Hippocampal control of the activity of thalamic neurones. *Helv. Physiol. Acta*, 1964, 22 : 28.

MARON, LOUISE, RECHTSCHAFFEN, A., and WOLPERT, E. A. The sleep cycle during napping. *Arch. Gen. Psychiat.*, 1964, 11 : 503–508.

MATHIS, J. L. PIERCE, C. M., and LESTER, B. K. Biochemical studies of sleep and dreams. APSS, 1962, Chicago.

MATSUMOTO, J. and JOUVET, M. Effet de reserpine, DOPA et 5 HTP, sur les deux estats de sommeil. *Comptes rendus des seances de la Societe de Biologie*, 1964, 158 : 2037.

MATSUZAKI, M., TAKAGI, H., TOKIZANE, T. Paradoxical phase of sleep : its artificial induction in the cat by sodium butyrate. *Science*, 1964, 146 : 1328–1329.

McKENZIE, R. B. HARTMAN, B., and GRAVELINE, B. E. An exploratory study of sleep characteristics in a hypodynamic environment. Brooks Air Force Base, Tex.: School of Aviation Medicine, 1960.

MEIER, G. W., and BERGER, R. J. The development of sleep and wakefulness patterns in the infant rhesus monkey. APSS, 1965, Washington, D.C.

MICHEL, F., JEANNEROD, M., MOURET, J., RECHTSCHAFFEN, A., and JOUVET, M. Sur les mechanismes de l'activite des pointes au niveau du systeme visuel au cours de la phase paradoxiale du sommeil. *C.R. Soc. Biol.*, 1964, 158 : 103–106.

MICHEL, F. KLEIN, M., JOUVET, DANIELLE, and VALATX, J. L. Etude polygraphique du sommeil chez le rat. *C.R. Soc. Biol.* In press.

MICHEL, F., RECHTSCHAFFEN, A., and VIMONT-VICARY, P., Activite electrique de muscles oculaires extrinseques au cours du cycle vielle-sommeil. *C.R. Soc. Biol.* 1964, 158 : 106–109.

MIKITEN, T. M., NIEBYL, P. H., and HENDLEY, C. D. EEG desynchronization during behavioral sleep associated with spike discharges from the thalamus of the cat. *Fed. Proc.*, 1960, 20 : 327.

MILLER, N. E. Chemical coding of behavior in the brain. *Science*, 1965, 148 : 328–338.

341

MIRSKY, A. F., and KORNETSKY, C. On the dissimilar effects of drugs on the digit symbol substitution and continuous performance tests: A review and preliminary integration of behavioral and physiological evidence. *Psychopharmacologia*, 1964. 5: 161–177.

MONNIER, M. Moderating brain stem systems inducing synchronization of the neocortex and sleep. *EEG Clin. Neurophysiol.*, 1962. 14: 426.

MONNIER, M., and HOSLI, L. Dialysis of sleep and waking factors in blood of the rabbit. *Science*, 1964, 146: 796–797.

MONROE, L. J. Psychological and physiological differences between good and poor sleepers. APSS, 1965, Washington, D.C. Unpublished doctoral dissertation, University of Chicago, 1965.

MONROE, L. J., RECHTSCHAFFEN, A., FOULKES, D., and JENSEN, JUDITH. The discriminability of REM and NREM reports. *J. Pers. Soc. Psychol.* In press.

MOORE, G. P., SEGUNDO, J. P., and PERKEL, D. H. Stability patterns in interneuronal pacemaker regulation. San Diego Symposium for Biomedical Engineering, 1963.

MORRIS, G. O., and SINGER, M. T. Sleep deprivation. *Arch. Gen. Psychiat.*, 1961, 5: 453.

MORUZZI, G. Active processes in the brain stem during sleep. *The Harvey Lecture Series*, 58. New York: Academic Press, 1962.

MORUZZI, G. The physiology of sleep. *Endeavour*, 1963, 22: 31–36.

MORUZZI, G. Reticular influences on the EEG. *EEG Clin. Neurophysiol.*, 1964, 16: 2–17.

MOURET, J. Les Mouvements Oculaires au cours du sommeil paradoxical. J. Tixier & Fils, 1964.

MURAWSKI, B. J., and CRABBE, J. Effect of sleep deprivation on plasma 17-hydroxycorticosteroids. *J. Appl. Physiol.*, 1960, 15: 280–282.

MURRAY, E. *Sleep, Dreams and Arousal.* New York: Appleton Century Crofts. In press.

MURRAY, E. J., SOHEIN, E. H., ERIKSON, K. T., HILL, W. F., and COHEN, M. The effects of sleep deprivation on social behavior. *J. Soc. Psych.*, 1959, 49: 229.

MURRAY, E. J., WILLIAMS, H. L. and LUBIN, A. Body temperature and psychological ratings during sleep deprivation. *J. Exp. Psych.*, 1958, 56.

MUZIO, J., ROFFWARG, H., and KAUFMAN, R. Alteration in the young adult human sleep EEG configuration resulting from d-LSD-25. APSS, 1964, Palo Alto.

O'CONNELL, D. N., and ORNE, M. T. Bioelectric correlates of hypnosis: an experimental reevaluation. *Psychiat. Res.*, 1962, 1: 201–213.

OFFENKRANTZ, W., and RECHTSCHAFFEN, A. Clinical studies of sequential dreams. I. A patient in psychotherapy. *Arch. Gen. Psychiat.*, 1963, 8: 497-508.

OFFENKRANTZ, W., and WOLPERT. E. The detection of dreaming in a congenitally blind subject. *J. Nerv. Ment. Dis.*, 1963, 136: 88–90.

ONHEIBER, PHYLLIS, WHITE, P., DeMYER, MARIAN K., and OTTINGER, D. Preliminary observations on the sleep and dreaming patterns of childhood schizophrenics. APSS, 1964, Palo Alto.

OSWALD, I. *Sleeping and Waking.* New York: Elsevier, 1962.

OSWALD, I., BERGER, R. J., JARAMILLO, R. A., KEDDIE, K. M. G., OLLEY, P. D., and PLUNKETT, G. B. Melancholia and barbiturates: a controlled EEG, body, and eye-movement study of sleep. *Brit. J. Psychiat.*, 1963 109: 66–78.

OSWALD, I., TAYLOR, A. M., and TREISMAN, M. Discriminative responses to stimulation during human sleep. *Brain*, 1960, 82: 440–453.

OSWALD, I., TAYLOR, A. M., and TREISMAN, M. Cortical function during human sleep. In *The Nature of Sleep.* Boston: Little, Brown, 1961, 343–348.

PAMPIGLIONE, B., and ACKNER, B. The effects of repeated stimulation upon EEG and vasomotor activity during sleep in man. *Brain*, 1958, 81: 64–75.

PARMEGGIANI, P. L., Hippocampal theta rhythm and neocortical responses to photic stimuli. *Helv. Physiol. Pharm. Acta.*, 1962, 20: 71.

PARMEGGIANI, P. L. Sincronizzazione dell "attivita bio-electrica dell" "ippocampo e resposta dell" area cerebrale primaria di proiezione acustica. *Arch. Sci. biol.*, 1962, 46: 121.

PARMEGGIANI, P. L., and ZANOCCO, G. A study on the bioelectrical rhythms of cortical and subcortical structures during activated sleep. *Arch. Ital. Biol.*, 1963, 101: 385.

PARMELEE, A. H. Sleep patterns in infancy. A study of one infant from birth to 8 months of age. *Acta Paediatrica*, 1961, 50: 160–170.

PARMELEE, A. H., AKIYAMA, Y., WENNER, W., and FLESCHER, JENNY. Activated sleep in premature infants. APSS, 1964, Palo Alto.

PARMELEE, A. H., SCHULZ, H. R., and DISBROW, M. A. Sleep patterns of the newborn. *J. Pediat.*, 1961, 58: 241.

PARMELEE, A. H., and WENNER, W. H. Sleep states in premature and full term newborn infants. APSS, 1965, Washington, D.C.

PARMELEE, A. H., WENNER, W. H., and SCHULZ, H. R. Infant sleep patterns: from birth to 16 weeks of age. *J. Pediat.*, 1964, 65: 576.

PASSEY, G. E., ALLUISI, E. A., and CHILES, W. D. Use of the experimental method for evaluations of performance in multi-man systems. Aerospace Medical Research Laboratories Memorandum, p. 67, 1964.

PASSOUANT, P., and CADILHAC, J. Les rhythmes theta hippocampique au cours du sommeil. In P. Passouant (ed.), *Physiologie de l'hippocampe*. Paris: Editions du C.N.R.S., 1962, 107: 331–347.

PEARLMAN, C., and GREENBERG, R. M. Relation of dreaming to formation of the memory trace. APSS, 1965, Washington, D.C.

PETSCHE, H., STUMPF, C., and GOGOLAK, G. The significance of the rabbit's septum as a relay station between the midbrain and the hippocampus. *EEG. Clin. Neurophysiol.*, 1962, 14: 202.

PIERCE, C. M., MATHIS, J. L., and JABBOUR, J. T. Dream patterns in narcoleptic and hydranencephalic patients. *Amer. Psychiat. Assn.*, New York, 1965.

PIERCE, C. M., WHITMAN, R. R., Maas, J. W., and GAY, M. I. Enuresis and dreaming. *Arch. Gen. Psychiat.*, 1961, 4: 166–170.

PIERCE, C. M., WHITMAN, R. R., MAAS, J. W., and GAY, M. I. Enuresis and dreaming. *Experimental Studies*, 1963.

PIZZARELLO, D. J., ISAAK, D., CHUA, K. E., and RHYNE, A. L. Circadian rhythmicity in the sensitivity of two strains of mice to whole-body radiation. *Science*, 1964, 145: 286–291.

POLLACK, C., WEITZMAN, E., and KRIPKE, D., Behavioral arousal thesholds during different sleep stages of the macaca mulatta. APSS, 1964, Palo Alto.

POND, A. Narcolepsy: A brief critical review and study of eight cases. *J. Ment. Sci.*, 1952, 98: 595–604.

PORTNOFF, G., BAEKLAND, F., GOODENOUGH, D. R., KARACAN, I., and SHAPIRO, A. The effect of sleep on retention. APSS, 1965, Washington, D.C.

RAND, R. W., CRANDALL, P. H., ADEY, W. R., WALTER, R. D., and MARKHAM, C. H. Electrophysiologic investigations in Parkinson's disease and other dyskinesias in man. *Neurology*, 1962, 12: 754–770.

RASMUSSEN, T. and PENFIELD, W. Movement of head and eyes from stimulation of the human frontal cortex. *Ass. Res. nerv. Dis. Proc.*, 1948, 27: 346.

RAY, J. T., MARTIN, O. E. and ALLUISI, E. A. Human performance as a function of the work-rest cycle. National Academy of Sciences-National Research Council, 1961. No. 882.

RECHTSCHAFFEN, A. Discussion of Dr. William Dement's paper "Experimental dream studies." *Science and psychoanalysis: Scientific proceedings of the Academy of Psychoanalysis*, vol. VII, New York, Grune & Stratton, 1964, pp. 162–170.

RECHTSCHAFFEN, A., CORNWALL, P., and ZIMMERMAN, W. Brain temperature variations with paradoxical sleep in the cat. APSS, 1965, Washington, D.C.

RECHTSCHAFFEN, A., and FOULKES, D. The effect of visual stimuli on dream content. *Percept. Mot. Skills*, 1965, 20: 149–1160.

345

RECHTSCHAFFEN, A., GOODENOUGH, D. R., and SHAPIRO, A. Patterns of sleep talking. *Arch. Gen. Psychiat.*, 1962, 7: 418–426.

RECHTSCHAFFEN, A., and MARON, LOUISE. The effect of amphetamine on the sleep cycle. *EEG Clin. Neurophysiol.*, 1964, 16: 433–445.

RECHTSCHAFFEN, A., SCHULSINGER, F., and MEDNICK, S. Schizophrenia and physiological indices of dreaming. *Arch. Gen. Psychiat.*, 1964, 10: 89–93.

RECHTSCHAFFEN, A., and VERDONE, P. Amount of dreaming: Effect of incentive, adaptation to laboratory, and individual differences. *Percept. Mot. Skills*, 1964, 19: 947–958.

RECHTSCHAFFEN, A., VERDONE, P., and WHEATON, JOY. Reports of mental activity during sleep. *Canad. Psychiat. Assn. J.*, 1963, 8: 409–414.

RECHTSCHAFFEN, A., VOGEL, G., and SHAIKUN, G. Interrelatedness of mental activity during sleep. *Arch. Gen. Psychiat.*, 1963, 9: 536–547.

RECHTSCHAFFEN, A., WOLPERT, E. A., DEMENT W. C., MITCHELL, S. A., and FISHER, C. Nocturnal sleep of narcoleptics. *EEG Clin. Neurophysiol.*, 1963, 15: 599–609.

REDING, G. R., RUBRIGHT, W. C., RECHTSCHAFFEN, A., and DANIELS, R. S. Sleep pattern of tooth-grinding: its relationship to dreaming. *Science*, 1964, 145: 725–726.

REITE, M., ADEY, W. R., KAVAN, EVA, and RHODES, J., Electrophysiological correlates of sleep in the monkey. APSS, 1964, Palo Alto.

RHODES, J. M. Sleep in the chimpanzee. APSS, 1964, Palo Alto.

RHODES, J. M., REITE, H. L., BROWN, D., and ADEY, W. R. Cortical and subcortical relationships in the chimpanzee during different phases of sleep. *Neurophysiologie des etats de sommeil*, Editions du Centre National de la Recherche Scientifique, Paris, 1965.

RICHTER, C. P. *Biological Clocks in Medicine and Psychiatry.* Charles C. Thomas, 1965.

RICKLES, W. H. A physiological study of sleep in the immature chimpanzee. APSS, 1965, Washington, D.C.

346

RISER, L., and LEVEY, J., et al. Influence de la serotonine et du 5 HTP sur le sommeil experimental en presence ou non d'iproniazide. *Rev. Agressologie*, 1960, 1: 4.

RISER, M., LABOUCARIE, J. De certains aspects du somnambulisme. *Toulouse Med. J.*, 1962, 4: 429–434.

ROFFWARG, H. P., DEMENT, W. C., and FISHER, C. Preliminary observations on the sleep-dream patterns in neonates, infants, children, and adults. In E. Harms (ed.), *Problems of Sleep and Dreams in Children*. London: Pergamon, 1963.

ROFFWARG, H. P., DEMENT, W. C., MUZIO, J. N., and FISHER, C. Dream imagery: relationship to rapid eye movements of sleep. *Arch. Gen. Psychiat.*, 1962, 7: 235–258.

ROFFWARG, H. P., MUZIO, J. N., and DEMENT, W. C. Ontogentic Development of the Human Sleep-Dream Cycle. *Science*, in press.

ROLDAN, E., WEISS, T., and FIFKOVA, E. Excitability changes during the sleep cycle of the rat. *EEG Clin. Neurophysiol.*, 1963, 15: 775–785.

ROSNER, B. S., GOFF, W. R. ALLISON, T. Cerebral electrical responses to external stimuli. In *EEG and Behavior*, G. H. Glasser (ed.), 1963, New York Basic Books.

ROSS, J. Neurological findings after prolonged sleep deprivation. APSS. 1964, Palo Alto.

ROSSI, G. F. Sleep-inducing mechanisms in the brain stem. *EEG Clin. Neurophysiol.*, 1962, 14: 428.

ROSSI, G. F., CANDIA, O., and MINOBE, K. Experimental findings on the anatomical location of the brain structures responsible for the deepest stage of sleep in the cat. APSS, 1963, New York.

ROSSI, G. F., FAVALE, E., HARA, T., GIUSSANI, A., and SACCO, G. Researches on the nervous mechanisms underlying deep sleep in the cat. *Arch. Ital. Biol.*, 1961, 99: 270–292.

ROTH, B. The clinical and theoretical importance of EEG rhythms corresponding to states of lowered vigilance. *EEG Clin. Neurophysiol.*, 1961, 13: 395–399.

SAINT-LAURENT, J., BATINI, C., BROUGHTON, P. and GAS-
TAUT, H. A polygraphic study of nocturnal enuresis in
the epileptic child. *EEG Clin. Neurophysiol.*, 1963, 15:
904.

SAMPSON, H. The laboratory dream. APSS, 1965, Washington, D.C.

SAMPSON, H. Deprivation of dreaming sleep by two
methods. APSS, 1965, Washington, D.C.

SAWYER, C. H. Some effects of sex hormones on brain
function. Proceedings of Third World Congress of
Psychiatry, University of Toronto Press, 1961, 118–120.

SAWYER, C. H. Mechanisms by which drugs and hormones activate and block release of pituitary gonado-
tropins. Proceedings of First International Pharmaco-
logical Meeting, vol. I, Pergamon Press, 1963, 27–46.

SAWYER, C. H., and KAWAKAMI, M. Characteristics of behavioral and electro-encephalographic after-reactions to
copulation and vaginal stimulation in the female rabbit. *Endocrinology*, 1959, 622–630.

SAWYER, C. H., and KAWAKAMI, M. Interactions between
the central nervous system and hormones influencing
ovulation. In C. A. Villee (ed.), *Control of Ovulation.*
Pergamon Press, 1961.

SAWYER, C. H., KAWAKAMI, M., MARKEE, J. E., and EVER-
ETT, J. M. Physiological studies on some interactions
between the brain and the pituitary-gonad axis in the
rabbit. *Endocrinology*, 1959, 65: 614–688.

SCHEIBEL, MADGE E., and SCHEIBEL, A. B. Some struc-
turo-functional correlates of development in young cats.
EEG Clin. Neurophysiol., 1963, supp. 24, 235.

SCHEIBEL, MADGE E., and SCHEIBEL, A. B. Some neural
substrates of postnatal development. *First Annual Review of Child Development.* M. Hoffman (ed.). In
press.

SCHEIN, E. H. The effects of sleep deprivation on performance in a simulated communication task. *J. Appl.
Psych.*, 1957, 41.

SCHWARTZ, BETTY A., GUILBAUD, G., and FISCHGOLD, H.
Single and multiple spikes in the night sleep of epileptics. *EEG Clin. Neurophysiol.*, 1964, 16: 56–67.

SCOTT, J. Blood plasma free fatty acid levels during sleep. APSS, 1964, Palo Alto.

SCOTT, J. Sleep patterns in normal and enuretic children (4–16 years). APSS, 1964, Palo Alto.

SCOTT, J. Sleeping and dreaming in enuretic children. APSS, 1964, Palo Alto.

SEGUNDO, J. P. A hypothesis concerning the sharp pitch discrimination observed in the sleeping cat. *Experientia.*, 1964, 20: 415.

SEGUNDO, J. P., MOORE, G. P., STENSAAS, L. J., and BULLOCK, T. H. Sensitivity of neurones in *Aplysia* to temporal pattern of arriving impulses. *J. Exp. Biol.*, 1963, 40: 643–667.

SEMAGIN, V. N. Sleep in the Arctic. *Fiziol. zh. ssr. Sechenov.*, 1961, 47: 8–11.

SHAPIRO, A. A comparison of the electrical activity recorded from the scalp with that recorded from various parts of the brain during spontaneous nocturnal sleep in a human subject. APSS, 1962, Chicago.

SHAPIRO, A., GOODENOUGH, D. R., BIEDERMAN, I., and SLESER, I. Dream recall and the physiology of sleep. *J. App. Physiol.*, 1964, 19.

SHAPIRO, A., GOODENOUGH, D. R., and GRYLER, R. B. Dream recall as a function of method of awakening. *Psychosom. Med.*, 1963, 25: 174–180.

SHEVRIN, H. and LUBORSKY, L. The measurement of preconscious preception in dreams and images: An investigation of the Poetzl phenomenon. *J. Abnorm. Soc. Psych.*, 1958, 56: 285–294.

SHNEIDMAN, E. S. Suicide, sleep, and death: some possible interrelations among cessation, interruption, and continuation phenomena. *Review*, 1963.

SIMON, C. W. Repetitive verbal stimulation during drowsy states as a technique for learning and problem solving, and the modification of human behavior and attitudes. *Hughes Aircraft*, 1961.

SIMON, C. W. Some immediate effects of drowsiness and sleep on normal human performance. *Human Factors*, 1961, 3.

SIMON, C. W., and EMMONS, W. H. Learning during sleep. *Psychol. Bull.*, 1955, 52: 328–342.

SIMON, C. W., and EMMONS, W. H. EEG, consciousness, and sleep. *Science*, 1956, 124: 1066–1069.

SIMON, C. W., and EMMONS, W. H. Responses to material presented during various levels of sleep. *J. Exp. Psychol.*, 1956, 51: 89–97.

SMELIK, P. G., and SAWYER, C. H. Effects of implantation of cortisol into the brain stem of pituitary gland on the adrenal response to stress in the rabbit. *Acta Endocrinol.*, 1962, 41: 561–570.

SMITH, F., and HALL, C. S. An investigation of regression in a long dream series. *J. Gerontol.*, 1964.

SNYDER, F. Dream recall, respiratory variability and depth of sleep. Address, Symposium on Dreams, *Amer. Psychiat. Assn.*, 1960.

SNYDER, F. Autonomic concomitants of REM and NREM sleep. APSS, 1962, Chicago.

SNYDER, F. The new biology of dreaming. *Arch. Gen. Psychiat.*, 1963, 8: 381–391.

SNYDER, F. The REM state in a living fossil. APSS, 1964, Palo Alto.

SNYDER, F. Progress in the new biology of dreaming. *Am. Psychiat. Assn.*, 1965, New York.

SNYDER, F. The organismic state associated with dreaming. In N. S. Greenfield and W. C. Lewis (eds.), *Psychoanalysis and Current Biological Thought*. University of Wisconsin Press, 1965, 275–315.

SNYDER, F., HOBSON, J. A., and GOLDFRANK, F. Blood pressure changes during human sleep. *Science*, 1963, 142: 1313–1314.

SNYDER, F., HOBSON, J. A., MORRISON, D. R., and GOLD-FRANK, F. Changes in respiration, heart rate, and systolic blood pressure in human sleep. *J. Appl. Physiol.*, 1964, 19: 417–422.

STERMAN, M. B., and CLEMENTE, C. D. Forebrain inhibitory mechanisms: Cortical synchronization induced by basal forebrain stimulation. *Exp. Neurol.*, 1962, 6: 91–102.

STERMAN, M., KNAUSS, T., LEHMANN, D., and CLEMENTE, C. Sleep and waking in the isolated cat: Effects of basal forebrain lesions. APSS, 1964, Palo Alto.

STOYVA, J. The effect of suggested dreams on the length of rapid eye movement periods. APSS, 1962, Chicago.

STOYVA, J., KAMIYA, J., and FORSYTH, R. Observations of blood pressure and heart rate in the sleeping macaca mulatta. APSS, 1965, Washington, D.C.

SUZUKI, I. Effects of insufficient sleep on serum cholesterol and blood reduced rutathione level. *Rodo Kagaku*, 1961, 37: 166.

TART, C. T. Frequency of dream recall and some personality measures. *J. Consult. Psychol.*, 1962, 26: 467–470.

TART, C. T. Effects of posthypnotic suggestion on the process of dreaming. Unpublished doctoral dissertation, University of North Carolina, 1963.

TART, C. T. A comparison of suggested dreams occurring in hypnosis and sleep. *Inter. J. Clin. Exp. Hypnosis*, 1964, 12: 263–389.

TROSMAN, H. RECHTSCHAFFEN A., OFFENKRANTZ, W., and WOLPERT, E. A. Studies in psychophysiology of dreams. IV. Relations among dreams in sequence. *Arch. Gen. Psychiat.*, 1960, 3: 602–607.

TYLER, F. M., MIGEON, C., FLORENTIN, A. A., and SAMUELS, L. T. The diurnal variation of 17-hydroxycorticosteroid levels in plasma. *J. Clin. Endocrinol.*, 1954, 14: 774.

VALATX, J. L., JOUVET, D., and JOUVET, M. Evolution electroencephalographique des differents estats de sommeil chez le chaton. *EEG Clin. Neurophysiol.*, 1964, 17: 218–233.

VALLEALA, P., and EVARTS, E. V. The temporal relation of unit discharge in visual cortex and activity of the extraocular muscles during sleep. APSS, 1965, Washington, D.C.

VAUGHN, C. J. The development and use of an operant technique to provide evidence for visual imagery in the rhesus monkey under "sensory deprivation." Doctoral dissertation, University of Pittsburgh, 1964.

VELLUTI, R., and HERNANDEZ-PEON, R. Atropine blockade within a cholinergic hypnogenic circuit. *Exp. Neurol.*, 1963, 8: 20–29.

VERDONE, P. P. Variables related to the temporal reference of manifest dream content. *Percept. Mot. Skills*, 1965, 20: 1253–1268.

VOGEL, G. Studies in psychophysiology of dreams. III. The dream of narcolepsy. *Arch. Gen. Psychiat.*, 1960, 8: 421–428.

VONEULER, C., and GREEN, J. D. Excitation, inhibition and rhythmical activity in hippocampal pyramidal cells in rabbit. *Acta Physiol. Scand.*, 1960, 48: 110.

WEBB, WILSE B. Antecedents of sleep. *J. Exp. Psychol.*, 1957, 53: 162–166.

WEBB, WILSE B. An overview of sleep as an experimental variable (1940-59). *Science*, 1961, 134: 1421.

WEBB, WILSE B. Sleep deprivation: Age and exhaustion time in the rat. *Science*, 1962, 136: 1122.

WEBB, WILSE B. Some effects of prolonged sleep deprivation on the hooded rat. *J. Physiol. Comp. Psychol.*, 1962, 55: 791–793.

WEBB, WILSE B., and ADES, H. Sleep tendencies: Effects of barometric pressure. *Science*, 1964, 132: 263–264.

WEBB, WILSE B., and AGNEW, H. W. Reaction time and social response efficiency on arousal from sleep. *Percept. Mot. Skills*, 1964, 18: 783–784.

WEBB, WILSE B., and AGNEW, H. W. The results of continued partial sleep deprivation. APSS, 1965, Washington, D.C.

WEBB, WILSE B., and JEANNERET, P. R. Strength of grip on arousal from full night's sleep. *Percept. Mot. Skills*, 1963, 17: 759–761.

WEBB, WILSE B., and STONE S. A note on the sleep responses of young college adults. *Percept. Mot. Skills*, 1963, 16: 162.

WEINBERGER, N. M., and LINDSLEY, D. B. Behavioral and electroencephalographic arousal to contrasting novel stimulation. *Science*, 1964, 144: 1355–1357.

WEISS, T. Sleep cycle in rodents. APSS, 1964, Palo Alto.

WEITZMAN, E. D. A note on the EEG and eye movements during behavioral sleep in monkeys. *EEG Clin. Neurophysiol.*, 1961, 13: 790–794.

WEITZMAN, E. D., FISHBEIN, W., and GRAZIANI, L. Auditory evoked responses obtained from scalp of the full term new-born human during sleep. *Pediatrics*, 1965, 35: 458–462.

WEITZMAN, E. D., and KREMEN, H. Auditory evoked responses during different stages of sleep in man. *EEG Clin. Neurophysiol.*, 1965, 18: 65–70.

WEITZMAN, E. D., KRIPKE, D., and POLLAK, C. Cyclic activity in sleep of macaca mulatta. *Arch. of Neurol.*, 1965, 12: 463–467.

WEITZMAN, E. D., SCHAUMBERG, H., and FISHBEIN, W. Plasma 17-hydroxycorticosteroid levels during sleep in man. APSS, 1965, Washington, D.C.

WEST, L. J. United States Air Force prisoners of Chinese Communists. In *Methods of forceful indoctrination: observations and interviews*. Group for Advancement of Psychiatry Symposium, 1957, 4: 270–284.

WEST, L. J. A general theory of hallucinations and dreams. In L. J. West (ed.), *Hallucinations*. New York: Grune & Stratton, 1962.

WEST, L. J., JANSZEN, H. H., LESTER, B. K., and CORNELISOON, F. S. The psychosis of sleep deprivation. *Ann. N.Y. Acad. Sci.*, 1962, 96: 66–70.

WHITMAN, R. M. Drugs, dreams, and the experimental subject. *Canad. Psychiat. Assn., J.*, 1963, 8: 395–399.

WHITMAN, R. M. Remembering and forgetting dreams in psychoanalysis. *J. Amer. Psychoanal. Assn.*, 1963, 7: 752–774.

WHITMAN, R. M., ORNSTEIN, P., KRAMER, M., and BALDRIDGE, B. Hypnotic conflict implantation and dream formation. APSS, 1963, New York.

353

WHITMAN, R. M., PIERCE, C. M., and MAAS, J. Drugs and dreams. In L. Uhr and J. G. Miller (eds.), *Drugs and Behavior.* New York: Wiley, 1960.

WHITMAN, R. M., PIERCE, C. M., MAAS, J., and BALDRIDGE, B. Drugs and dreams. II. Imipramine and prochlorperazine. *Comp. Psychiat.*, 1961, 2: 219–226.

WHITMAN, R., PIERCE, C., MAAS, J., and BALDRIDGE, B. The dreams of the experimental subject. *J. Nerv. Ment. Dis.*, 1962, 134: 431–439.

WILKINSON, R. T. Muscle tension during mental work under sleep deprivation. *J. Exp. Psychol.*, 1962, 64: 565–571.

WILKINSON, R. T. Interaction of noise with knowledge of results and sleep deprivation. *J. Exp. Psychol.*, 1963, 66: 332–337.

WILKINSON, R. T. After effect of sleep deprivation. *J. Exp. Psychol.*, 1963, 66: 439–444.

WILKINSON, R. T. Effects of up to 60 hours of sleep deprivation on different types of work. *Ergonomics*, 1964, 7: 175–186.

WILKINSON, R. T. A review of sleep deprivation. In Edholme and Bacharach, (eds.), *The Physiology of Human Survival.* New York, Academic Press. In press.

WILLIAMS, H. L., GRANDA, A. M., JONES, R. C., LUBIN, A., and ARMINGTON, J. C. EEG frequency and finger pulse volume as predictors of reaction time during sleep loss. *EEG Clin. Neurophysiol.*, 1962, 14: 64–70.

WILLIAMS, H. L., HAMMACK, J. T., DALY, R. L., DEMENT, W. C., and LUBIN, A. Responses to auditory stimulation, sleep loss, and the EEG stages of sleep. *EEG Clin. Neurophysiol.*, 1964, 16: 269–279.

WILLIAMS, H. L., LUBIN, A., and GOODNOW, J. J. Impaired performance with acute sleep loss. *Psych. Monographs*, 73, No. 14.

WILLIAMS, H. L., MORLOCK, H. C., and MORLOCK, JEAN V. Discriminative responses to auditory signals during sleep. APA, 1963, Philadelphia.

WILLIAMS, H. L., MORRIS, G. O., and LUBIN, A. Illusions, hallucinations, and sleep loss. In L. J. West (ed.), *Hallucinations.* New York: Grune & Stratton, 1962.

WILLIAMS, H. L., TEPAS, D. I., and MORLOCK, H. C. Evoked responses to clicks and electroencephalographic stages of sleep in man. *Science*, 1962, 138: 685–686.

WILLIAMS, R. L., AGNEW, H. W., and WEBB, WILSE B. Sleep patterns in young adults: an EEG study. *EEG Clin. Neurophysiol.*, 1964, 17: 376–381.

WILSON, W. P., and ZUNG, W. K. Arousal threshold of males and females during sleep. 10th Annual Conference VA Cooperative Studies in Psychiatry, New Orleans, La., March 1965.

WITKIN, H. A., and LEWIS, HELEN B. The relation of experimentally induced pre-sleep experiences to dreams: preliminary report. January 1964.

WOLPERT, E. A. Studies in psychophysiology of dreams. II. An electromyographic study of dreaming. *Arch. Gen. Psychiat.*, 1960, 2: 231–241.

WOLPERT, E. A., and TROSMAN, H. Studies in psychophysiology of dreams. I. Experimental evocation of sequential dream episodes. *Arch. Neurol. Psychiat.*, 1958, 79: 603–606.

WOLSTENHOLME, G. E. W., and O'CONNOR, M. (eds.), *The Nature of Sleep*. Boston: Little, Brown, 1960.

WOODS, R. L. *The World of Dreams*. New York: Random House, 1947.

WYRWICKA, W., STERMAN, M. B., and CLEMENTE, C. D. Conditioning of induced electroencephalographic sleep patterns in the cat. *Science*, 1962, 137: 616–618.

YOKOTA, T., and FUJIMORI, B. Effects of brain-stem stimulation upon hippocampal electrical activity, somatomotor reflexes and autonomic functions. *The EEG Journal*, 1964, 16: 375:

YOKOTA, T., SATO, A., and FUJIMORI, B. Inhibition of sympathetic activity by stimulation of the limbic system. *Japan J. Physiol.*, 1963, 13: 138.

YOSS, R. E., and DALY, D. D. Criteria for the diagnosis of the narcoleptic syndrome. *Proc. Staff Meet. Mayo Clin.*, 1957, 32: 320–328.

YOSS, R. E., and DALY, D. D. Narcolepsy. *Arch. Int. Med.*, 1960, 106: 168–171.

Yoss, R. E, and DALY, D D. Narcolepsy in children. *Pediatrics*, 1960, 25 : 1025-1033.

Yoss, R. E., and DALY, D. D. Hereditary aspects of narcolepsy. *Trans. Amer. Neurol. Assn.*, 1960, 239–240.

ZANCHETTI,, A. Electroencephalographic activation during sleep after destruction of midbrain-limbic pathways in the cat. APSS, 1963, New York.

ZUNG, W. K., NAYLOR, T., GIANTURCO, D., and WILSON, W. P. Computer simulation of sleep EEG patterns using a Markov chain model, *Recent Advances in Biological Psychiatry*, vol. VIII, Plenum Press, New York, 1965.

ZUNG, W. K., and WILSON, W. P. Auditory stimuli discrimination during sleep. *EEG Clin. Neurophysiol.*, 1961, 13 : 313.

ZUNG, W. K., and WILSON, W. P. Response to auditory stimulation during sleep. *Arch. Gen. Psychiat.*, 1961, 4 : 548–552.

ZUNG, W. K., WILSON, W. P., and DODSON, W. E. Effect of depressive disorders on sleep EEG arousal. *Arch. Gen. Psychiat.*, 1964, 10 : 439.

Appendix

THE FOUR STAGES OF SLEEP

Only recently scientists have been able to analyze sleep. This was made possible by the invention of the electroencephalograph (EEG) -- a machine that can measure and record "brain waves" -- the brain's recurrent electrical patterns. The changes that these patterns undergo during sleep are recorded by the EEG for researchers to analyze. Based on such changes, scientists have divided sleep into four stages.

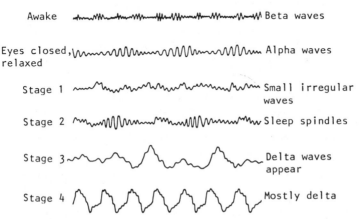

Changes in brain-wave patterns associated with various stages of sleep.

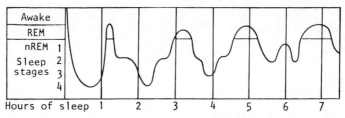

Typical changes in stages of sleep during the night.

Before actual sleep, a subject is in a relaxed waking state with his eyes closed. The EEG illustrates this state in the form of alpha brain waves or alpha rhythm, a wave pattern of 10 cycles per second. Sleep begins with the onset of Initial Stage 1 EEG. Here, the alpha rhythm is replaced by slower, irregular waves. However, this EEG pattern is not very different from that found in an active, awake person. As the individual falls further into sleep, the wave pattern increases to 14 cycles per second bringing the person into Stage 2 sleep. This stage is characterized by spindles -- sharply pointed waves recorded by the EEG. Larger and slower delta waves appear in Stage 3 of sleep. These waves measure one to two cycles per second. Both spindles and delta waves appear in Stage 3. However, in Stage 4, delta waves predominate. The entire cycle of Stages 1 through 4 is executed four to six times during an average eight hour period of sleep.

Another important stage of sleep is called Stage 1-REM. Eugene Aserinsky found that rapid eye movements (REM's) occur during Stage 1 EEG. These REM's are jerky movements of the eyes beneath the eyelids. REM's are detected and measured by a machine called an electroculogram (EOG). In his research, Aserinsky found that in about 80 percent of the time, subjects who were awakened during these periods reported a dream.

358

Dreams generally occur during this stage, although dreamlike activity can occur in other stages of sleep. The Stage 1-REM is a period of deep sleep even though its EEG pattern is similar to that of an active, awake individual. For this reason, it has been called "paradoxical sleep."

As each cycle of sleep is repeated, the Stage 1-REM becomes longer. The first one occurs about 90 minutes after sleep has begun and lasts for about 5 to 10 minutes. The stage increases in duration at each 90 minute cycle. As expected, the last Stage 1-REM stage is the longest. During this stage, the sleeper experiences the longest and most vivid dreams. A dream during this stage can last from half an hour to an hour This last dream is the one that is most likely to be recalled. Quite often, the individual awakens during the last Stage 1-REM.

THE HYPNOPOMPIC AND HYPNAGOGIC STATES

The hypnagogic state refers to the state one experiences when going from a wakeful state to sleep. This state is highly similar to the hypnopompic state, when one goes from sleep to wakefulness. Some researchers believe that the two states are practically identical.

The limited research in this area has focused on the hypnagogic state. The most recent studies have consisted of experiments in which subjects were awakened while they were in a hypnagogic state and asked to describe their experiences. Based on the subjects' reports, the hypnagogic state has been described in terms of three ego states: intact ego state, destructuralized ego state, and restructuralized ego state. In the intact ego state, the subject remains in contact with his external environment. He can control his mental processes and distinguish

359

between the internal and external world.   In the
intact ego state, the subject recognizes his location
in the outside world.   In the destructuralized ego

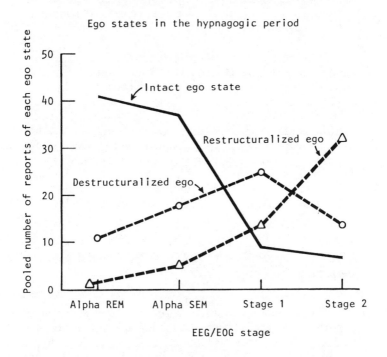

Ego states in the hypnagogic period

state, the subject loses contact with the external
world and a sense of his place in that world. Mental
content in this state is no longer reality-oriented. In
the restructuralized ego state, mental content is
relatively logical and reality-oriented but there is no
contact with the external environment.

Investigators have found that reports which
indicate the presence of intact ego states are
highest at the beginning of the hypnagogic period
-- at alpha rhythm. As sleep progresses, however,
the incidence of intact ego states decreases. The
number of reports of a decentralized ego state is

360

relatively low. The number increases through Stage 1 sleep, then declines at Stage 2 sleep. Very few reports of a restructuralized ego state occur at the beginning of the hypnagogic period, but they gradually increase throughout all stages of falling asleep.

From these results, a trend can be noted. Contact with the external environment is gradually lost as sleep begins and progresses. Mental content is at first logical, it then becomes bizarre and is followed by a stage that exhibits some logic in mental content despite the fact that there is no contact with the outside world.

THE EFFECTS OF SLEEP DEPRIVATION

A wide range of effects result from sleep deprivation. Behavioral changes after sleep deprivation can be as mild as simple irritability or as dramatic as bizarre hallucinations.

In a study conducted at UCLA (Pasnau, et al., 1968) four subjects were deprived of sleep for a period of 205 consecutive hours. The effects were both mild and dramatic. One subject, who experienced a very dramatic effect, became hysterical during a psychomotor training task and screamed incoherently upon hallucinating a gorilla.

Prolonged sleep deprivation -- 220 hours or more -- can lead to psychotic-like behavior. Studies have indicated that those who displayed this type of behavior often had traumatic childhoods and neurotic and work disturbances. Other physiological changes that occur as a result of sleep deprivation include a decrease in the amount of alpha brain waves and a low voltage EEG.

Dreaming occurs during the Stage 1-REM period

361

of sleep. Aserinsky and Kleitman (1953) reported incidents of increased heart rate and breathing during these periods of rapid eye movements. Other researchers have reported that the body's central nervous system is active during this period, undergoing severe fluctuations in heartbeat and blood pressure.

Studies have been conducted on REM deprivation in which subjects slept but were awakened each time they entered the REM period. A control group was also employed whose subjects were awakened the same number of times as the REM-deprived subjects, but only during non-REM periods. Researchers found that during each successive night of the experiment, the REM-deprived subjects entered into more REM periods. During the day, these subjects appeared more tense, irritable and generally more anxious than the control group subjects. The REM-deprived subjects experienced difficulty in concentrating and remembering. When the experimenters finally allowed the REM-deprived subjects to sleep without interruption, the sleepers dreamed 60 percent more than usual. This additional dreaming has been called "REM rebound."

These studies seem to indicate that man has a need to dream.

SOMNAMBULISM

Somnambulism, or sleepwalking as it is more commonly called, is reported to exist in 1 to 5 percent of the population. The incidence has been found to be high among males, children, and among those who have suffered from enuresis (bedwetting) and have had a family history of somnambulism.

Psychology offers several explanations for somnambulism. Some psychologists regard it as a dissociative state in which there is a loss of memory and awareness of identity. Others regard it as a dreamlike disturbance of consciousness. Because sleepwalking is more common in children than adults, it is often viewed as an immature habit pattern. If sleepwalking persists into adulthood a more severe diagnosis is applied.

Some researchers consider somnambulism as a symptom of an epileptic state. They have found that a higher frequency of EEG abnormalities occurs among sleepwalkers than non-sleepwalkers.

Psychologists share very different views on the actual condition of sleepwalking. Some psychologists report that it is a state in which the individual is not awake. Others describe it as a state in which the person is not asleep. Psychologists generally disagree about motor ability during this state. Psychologists generally agree that after he awakens, the sleepwalker experiences total amnesia for the somnambulistic incident. A single sleepwalking episode usually lasts approximately 15 to 30 minutes.

FREUD'S THEORY OF DREAMS

Sigmund Freud was the first major psychologist who considered dreams meaningful. Before Freud's development of psychoanalysis, psychologists believed that dreams consisted of either useless information or the refuse of mental life. Freud used dreams in the design of his psychoanalytic theory. He believed that dreams provide the clearest example of unconscious processes at work. According to psychoanalytic theory, the psychological energy one uses during waking periods is shifted both to the unconscious and to certain perceptual areas of the brain during sleep. When one begins to dream, the external world is almost completely eliminated and replaced by an internal world. The content of dreams is dependent upon the emotions that have been aroused during the previous day. These emotions are associated with the primary sex and aggression drives as well as the repressed memories that center on these drives.

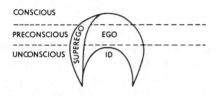

The Relationship of Personality Structures to the Levels of Awareness

Freud analyzed the dreams of both children and adults. He found that children's dreams often consist of wish fulfillment. These dreams deal with the wishes the child is aware of as well as those which are unconscious. A child who experiences an intense desire to own a particular toy, for example, might dream that he gets it.

In the dreams of adults, motives are not as clear. Although most adults report their dreams to be nonsensical and confused, Freud identified two types of interrelated dream content. First, there is the manifest content of the dream. This is the information about the dream that the individual remembers and can report. Beneath this surface content is a latent content. Latent content consists of unconscious desires which are usually related to the sex and aggression drives. Freud suggested that recognition of these wishes during waking hours may be too painful or unacceptable to consciousness Therefore, these wishes find expression through dreams.

Even in dreams, however, these unconscious

364

wishes are not expressed directly. Instead, they are expressed in disguised form through what Freud called the dream processes

Common Freudian dream interpretations and their symbols:

1. Parents- emperors, empresses, kings, queens
2. Children (brothers and sisters)- small animals
3. Birth- water
4. Death- journey
5. Nakedness- clothes, uniforms
6. Male genitals- sticks, umbrellas, poles, trees, anything elongated, pointed weapons of all sorts
7. Erection- balloons, airplanes, zeppelins, dreamer himself flying
8. Male sexual symbols- Reptiles, fishes, serpent, hand or foot
9. Female genitalia- pits, hollow caves, jars, bottles, doors, ships, chests
10. Breasts- apples, peaches, other fruit
11. Intercourse- mounting a ladder or stairs, entering a room, walking down a hall or into a tunnel, horseback riding, and so forth

In this way, the individual's conscience is not aroused.

Freud identified four dream processes by which unconscious desires are disguised in dreams. The first process is called condensation. Here, people and objects are represented with the characteristics of several different familiar individuals and objects. For example, a character in a dream may look like someone one knows, dress like another, speak like a third, and have the name of a fourth.

Freud identified the second dream process as displacement. Displacement involves a reallocation of psychic energy. The elements that figure most prominently in the manifest dream do not have much significance with regard to unconscious drives;

hence, they carry little psychic energy. Those elements that are replete with psychic energy are the small details in dreams. Often these details cannot be recalled.

The third dream process, symbolization, stemmed from Freud's observations that certain dream elements have common meanings for many people. However, most people cannot identify or interpret the latent meaning of these elements.

In the last dream process, secondary elaboration, dream elements are arranged in a certain order to form the whole dream. This process involves the incorporation of a story line or the use of events from the previous day to fill in transitions between the significant dream elements and unify the dream.

According to Freud, the major purpose of the dream processes is to arrange a compromise: to allow the dreamer gratification from unconscious drives yet keep them hidden from a repulsed conscience. Freud's theory is important because it challenged the myth that dreams are insignificant. However, his theory awaits proof. Most of its critics argue that it lacks a scientific method for the analysis of dream content.

To Freud dreams represented attempts at wish fulfillment. He reasoned that the dream is a hallucinatory state that structures events not as they would be in reality, but as the dreamer wishes them to be. When unconscious desires conflict with conscious restraints, however, it is necessary for the "dream work" to pursue devious paths to express the wish. Thus, Freud believed dreams to be an uncommonly rich source of unconscious material. He maintained that a skilled observer reviewing the contents of dreams could discover much useful information in the unconscious mind of the dreamer. Thus, Freud referred to dreams as "the royal road to the unconscious."

Because of the disguised nature of wish fulfillment in dreams, Freud distinguished between the
manifest content of a dream (the literal content of
the dream as experienced by the dreamer) and the
latent content (the hidden, symbolic, actual meaning
of the dream).

Dream Analysis

An infantile dream, recalled many years later, points
for Freud to the deep-seatedness and long-lasting-
ness of psychosexual experiences in the infant years.

> A man, now thirty-five, relates a clearly re-
> membered dream which he claims to have had
> when he was four years of age: The notary with
> whom his father's will was deposited--he had
> lost his father at the age of three--brought two
> large emperor pears, of which he was given one
> to eat. The other lay on the windowsill of the
> livingroom. He woke with the conviction of the
> reality of what he had dreamt, and obstinately
> asked his mother to give him the second pear; it
> was, he said, still lying on the windowsill. His
> mother laughed at this.

Freud says:

> The dreamer's inability to associate justifies the
> attempt to interpret it by the substitution of
> symbols. The two pears...are the breasts of the
> mother who nursed him; the windowsill is a
> projection of the bosom. His sensation of
> reality after waking is justified, for his mother
> had actually suckled him for much longer than
> the customary term, and her breast was still
> available. The dream is to be translated:
> "Mother, give me the breast again at which I

once used to drink." The "once" is represented by the eating of one pear, the "again" by the desire for the other.

JUNG'S THEORY OF DREAMS

Carl G. Jung, a Swiss physician, was one of the most outstanding critics of Freud's theory. He believed that it was too restrictive and that it neglected some important aspects of man's dreaming. According to Jung, certain dream elements are characteristic of all people. Jung believed that some underlying personal elements in a dream are common to all people, regardless of cultural and individual differences. These elements are archetypal; they are characteristic of man as a species. For example, if someone were to dream about climbing a mountain, Freud would see this dream as reflective of a past event or wish in the individual's life. Jung, however, would expand upon this interpretation to include a characteristic common to all people. In this case, it would be the desire for achievement, to rise to the top. Jung also believed that a person's personality in his dreams is the opposite of his personality when he is awake. For example, a person who is usually outspoken would be very timid in a dream.

Another non-Freudian theory about dreams holds that dreams are continuous or congruent with thoughts people have when they are awake. Many psychologists agree that problems people worry about while awake are usually the same problems they worry about in dreams. The same needs and desires apparent in wakefulness are also present in dreams. Psychologists have found that subjects who have been deprived of food report more dreams in which food is a major element than subjects in a control group. Hence, the theory that dreams continue the thoughts experienced in wakefulness is dissimilar to Jung's theory that dream thoughts are opposite to waking thoughts, and Freud's theory that dreams represent expressions of unconscious desires which are repulsive or disagreeable to consciousness.

DAYDREAMS

A daydream is a fantasy created by an individual during a waking state. In daydreams, a person conjures up images of scenes or events which are extremely gratifying. These images often reflect egoistic desires for power, prestige, wealth or erotic pleasures.

Daydreams are not related to dreams experienced during sleep. Daydreams do not share the same basic characteristics: their content is more closely related to reality and they are usually more logical and coherent. Hence, daydreams can be reported with more ease than dreams.

The important difference between daydreams and dreams is the element of control. Daydreams are controlled by one's waking consciousness, and one can determine the exact nature of the daydream. The mental images and processes are under control. In dreams the mind does not have this degree of control.

Furthermore, in a daydream, the healthy individual recognizes that he is fantasizing whereas in dreams, the individual does not realize that he is dreaming.

The mental processes that convert wishes and impulses into the disguised images of the manifest content are called the "dream work." It is the function of the psychoanalyst to interpret or undo this dream work, to unravel the manifest content and reveal the more fundamental latent content from which the dream was derived. The study and interpretation of dream imagery was one of Freud's major contributions to the study of the unconscious. He believed that a "censorship system" existed at the border of the conscious mind that was very selective about the impulses it would allow the dreamer to recall to his conscious mind. Wishes that would be morally unacceptable to the awake dreamer would not be allowed to appear undisguised in a dream. This distortion by the censorship system made possible the fulfillment of hidden wishes without too much disturbance to the dreamer. Thus, the only way that the unconscious could achieve satisfaction for its strong desires was by evading the censor by masquerading the unacceptability of its wishes behind the facade of neutral objects or ideas. It is the unconscious and the censor together, therefore, that are responsible for dream content and it is for this reason that their interpretation could contribute so much to the understanding of the dreamer's motivations.

Have you ever dreamed of . . . ?	%
1. being attacked or pursued	82.8
2. falling	77.2
3. trying again and again to do something	71.2
4. school, teachers, studying	71.2
5. being frozen with fright	58.0
6. sexual experiences	66.4
7. eating delicious food	61.6
8. falling with fear	67.6
9. arriving too late, e.g., missing train	63.6
10. fire	40.8
11. swimming	52.0
12. dead people as though alive	46.0
13. being locked up	56.4
14. loved person as dead	57.2
15. snakes	48.8
16. being on verge of falling	46.8
17. finding money	56.0
18. failing an examination	38.8
19. flying or soaring through air	33.6
20. being smothered, unable to breathe	44.4
21. falling without fear	33.2
22. wild, violent beasts	30.0
23. being inappropriately dressed	46.0
24. seeing self as dead	33.2
25. being nude	42.8
26. killing someone	25.6
27. being tied, unable to move	30.4
28. having superior knowledge or mental ability	25.6
29. lunatics or insane people	25.6
30. your teeth falling out	20.8
31. creatures, part animal, part human	14.8
32. being buried alive	14.8
33. seeing self in mirror	12.4
34. being hanged by neck	2.8

Percentage of college students who have experienced common dream themes.

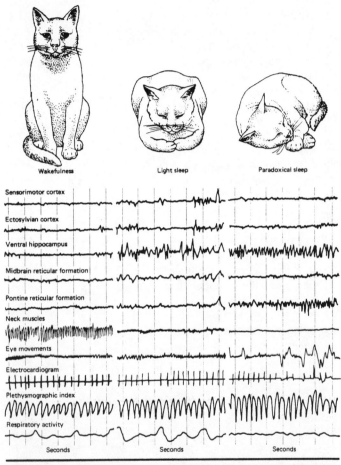

In cats, the characteristic bodily rhythms associated with deep sleep (the group of traces on the right) are so much like those of wakefulness (the group on the left) and so different from those of light sleep (the middle group) that the term "paradoxical" has been applied to deep sleep. Normally, cats sleep about two-thirds of the time. They usually begin a sleep period with 25 minutes of light sleep, followed by 6 or 7 minutes of "paradoxical" sleep. The electrical activity of brain structures and records of bodily activity during the three periods are also shown.

Ego States in the Hypnagogic Period

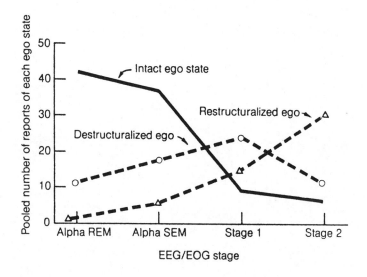

Reports of hypnagogic activity classified into different ego states as a function of brain wave activity (EEG) and eye movements (EOG) at the time of the report. Physiological tests states are alpha wave EEG with rapid eye movement (REM), alpha wave EEG with slow eye movement (SEM), Initial Stage 1 sleep (without REMs), and Stage 2 sleep.

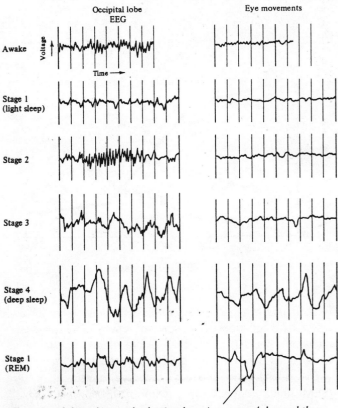

Occipital lobe EEG   Eye movements

Awake

Stage 1
(light sleep)

Stage 2

Stage 3

Stage 4
(deep sleep)

Stage 1
(REM)

Electroencephalographic records, showing the various stages of sleep and the record of eye movements that accompany them. Stage 1 (REM) resembles somewhat light sleep, but, as you can see, REM sleep is accompanied by eye movements, one of which is indicated by the arrow.
From Kleitman, 1960.